GLOBAL PUBLIC HEALTH AND FLUORIDE AS A VACCINE FOR TOOTH DECAY

THE 3RD MOST PREVALENT DISEASE IN THE WORLD AND ITS "VACCINE"

Editora Appris Ltda.
1.ª Edição - Copyright© 2025 dos autores
Direitos de Edição Reservados à Editora Appris Ltda.

Nenhuma parte desta obra poderá ser utilizada indevidamente, sem estar de acordo com a Lei nº
9.610/98. Se incorreções forem encontradas, serão de exclusiva responsabilidade de seus organi-
zadores. Foi realizado o Depósito Legal na Fundação Biblioteca Nacional, de acordo com as Leis nos
10.994, de 14/12/2004, e 12.192, de 14/01/2010.

Catalogação na Fonte
Elaborado por: Dayanne Leal Souza
Bibliotecária CRB 9/2162

N852g 2025	Noronha, Thiago Pompeu Global public health and fluoride as a vaccine for tooth decay: the 3rd most prevalent disease in the world and its "vaccine" / Thiago Pompeu Noronha, João Batista Filgueiras de Noronha. – 1. ed. – Curitiba: Appris, 2025. 91 p. ; 21 cm. – (General). Includes references. ISBN 978-65-250-7218-0 1. Vaccine. 2. Fluoride. 3. Tooth decay. I. Noronha, Thiago Pompeu. II. Noronha, João Batista Filgueiras de. III. Title. IV. Series. CDD – 614

Livro de acordo com a normalização técnica da ABNT

Appris
editorial

Editora e Livraria Appris Ltda.
Av. Manoel Ribas, 2265 – Mercês
Curitiba/PR – CEP: 80810-002
Tel. (41) 3156 - 4731
www.editoraappris.com.br

Printed in Brazil
Impresso no Brasil

Thiago Pompeu Noronha
João Batista Filgueiras de Noronha

GLOBAL PUBLIC HEALTH AND FLUORIDE AS A VACCINE FOR TOOTH DECAY

THE 3RD MOST PREVALENT DISEASE IN THE WORLD AND ITS "VACCINE"

Appris editora

Curitiba, PR
2025

FICHA TÉCNICA

EDITORIAL	Augusto Coelho Sara C. de Andrade Coelho

COMITÊ EDITORIAL

Ana El Achkar (Universo/RJ)
Andréa Barbosa Gouveia (UFPR)
Antonio Evangelista de Souza Netto (PUC-SP)
Belinda Cunha (UFPB)
Délton Winter de Carvalho (FMP)
Edson da Silva (UFVJM)
Eliete Correia dos Santos (UEPB)
Erineu Foerste (Ufes)
Fabiano Santos (UERJ-IESP)
Francinete Fernandes de Sousa (UEPB)
Francisco Carlos Duarte (PUCPR)
Francisco de Assis (Fiam-Faam-SP-Brasil)
Gláucia Figueiredo (UNIPAMPA/ UDELAR)
Jacques de Lima Ferreira (UNOESC)
Jean Carlos Gonçalves (UFPR)
José Wálter Nunes (UnB)
Junia de Vilhena (PUC-RIO)

Lucas Mesquita (UNILA)
Márcia Gonçalves (Unitau)
Maria Aparecida Barbosa (USP)
Maria Margarida de Andrade (Umack)
Marilda A. Behrens (PUCPR)
Marília Andrade Torales Campos (UFPR)
Marli Caetano
Patrícia L. Torres (PUCPR)
Paula Costa Mosca Macedo (UNIFESP)
Ramon Blanco (UNILA)
Roberta Ecleide Kelly (NEPE)
Roque Ismael da Costa Güllich (UFFS)
Sergio Gomes (UFRJ)
Tiago Gagliano Pinto Alberto (PUCPR)
Toni Reis (UP)
Valdomiro de Oliveira (UFPR)

SUPERVISORA EDITORIAL	Renata C. Lopes
PRODUÇÃO EDITORIAL	Daniela Nazário
REVISÃO	Bruna Fernanda Martins
DIAGRAMAÇÃO	Amélia Lopes
CAPA	Eneo Lage
REVISÃO DE PROVA	Jibril Keddeh

The more I learn, the more I realize how much I know nothing.
Knowledge is always infinite.

(Albert Einstein)

ACKNOWLEDGMENTS

To God, for the opportunity granted, for all the gifts and achievements provided and for those that will come to be realized, in this and other lives.

*To our beloved Noronha family: my wife, Bruna; and my son,
David, my parents, Ana and João; for all the support
and unconditional love today and always.*

LIST OF ABBREVIATIONS AND ACRONYMS

F - Fluorine

FA - Fluorapatite

HA - Hydroxyapatite

NaF - Sodium fluoride

WHO - World Health Organization

SUMÁRIO

1

INTRODUCTION 15

2

FLUORIDE 21

3

WHAT IS A VACCINE? 29

3.1 How Vaccines Work...29

3.2 Benefits of Vaccines 30

3.3 The ideal vaccine...30

3.4 Would fluoride as a vaccine be possible?..............................31

3.5 Fluoride as a vaccine against tooth decay in the world 32

3.6 Anti-cavity protocol and its vaccine.....................................32

3.7 Fluoride as a major modifier of quality of life and global health 34

4

LITERATURE REVIEW..37

4.1 Types of fluoride products 40

4.1.1 Fluoride Mouthwashes.. 40

4.1.2 Topical fluoride 42

4.1.3 Fluoridated water 45

4.1.4 Fluoridated toothpaste 49

4.1.5 Fluoride supplementation (tablets, tablets or medications) 52

4.1.6 Fluoride ingested in the diet 53

4.2 Creation of a global oral health campaign. Black March.......53

5

DISCUSSION..57

5.1 Controversy..58

5.2 Fluoride and its mode of action 65

5.3 Considerations on fluoride, health and oral infections not diagnosed by health professionals, which cause mortality in many patients 67

5.4 Oral Health and Undiagnosed Infections 67

5.5 Challenges in Detection and Diagnosis 68

5.6 Importance of Preventive Care 68

5.7 Protocol for the use of glass ionomer cement in caries 71

6

VOLUNTEER WORK AND DENTISTRY.......................75

6.1 Importance of Volunteering in Dentistry.................................75

7

CONCLUSION..81

REFERENCES 83

1

INTRODUCTION

A simple question to the noble reader of this book: have you ever had cavities? Have you ever had a toothache? If so, do you remember how painful it was? Have you ever had a root canal? Have you ever lost a tooth or more? Have you ever needed an implant? Do you use dentures? Did you spend a lot of money during the treatment? And if you could go back in time, would you like to change that reality? Can you imagine how much time and money you would save on this journey?

Would you like your children, grandchildren and great-grandchildren not to go through this?

If your answer was yes to any of these questions, you are in a position to change the reality not only of yourself but of the generations to come. In the context of the 3rd most common disease in the world, possibly the one that generates the most costs for both governments and citizens around the world (Noronha, Parente, 2024).

There has been a great evolution in recent decades regarding tooth loss. When compared to those born in the last century, a large proportion lost their teeth and had to use complete dentures, covering all the teeth in their mouth, causing many occlusal (bite) and TMJ (joint that connects the jaw to the skull) problems. In the next generation, of children, there was already a great improvement in the amount of cavities and lost teeth, while in the generation of their grandchildren there was another improvement, in which even fewer teeth were lost. However, all generations had cavities to a greater or lesser extent. Why did all this change occur?

It happened due to the use of fluoride and new technologies associated with brushing teeth with fluoride after meals, but this same generation of grandchildren still has cavities and often loses permanent teeth prematurely, today, in 2024. And there are ways to further mitigate these ills that bring health and socioeconomic problems to practically the entire world population, from the rich to the poor, from the 1st to the 3rd world, from the resident of Manhattan to the resident of the indigenous tribe in the Amazon. And this can and should be slowed down once and for all, if we create a simple protocol that is viable, when administered to the right age group, with the appropriate health education described and distributed to everyone.

The expanded concept of health, defined in article 196 of the Constitution of the Republic, should guide the progressive change of health services, evolving from a care model centered on disease and based on serving those who seek it, to a model of comprehensive health care, in which there is the progressive incorporation of promotion and protection actions, alongside those of recovery itself, in this way the most effective and cheapest way to prevent tooth decay is with the use of Fluoride and fluoride compounds (Brazil, 2004).

Dental caries is a complex disease resulting from many risk factors (Fejerskov, 2004). The prevalence of this disease has decreased in many countries around the world due to preventive measures. The main actions that have proven to be effective are: correct oral hygiene, dietary control and the use of fluorides. However, since the possibility of success of public health measures is related to complex cultural and behavioral problems, the decline in caries rates has been associated primarily with the action of fluorides (Murray, 1992).

The prevalence of tooth decay worldwide is high and continues to be a significant public health problem. According to the WHO, this disease is one of the most common diseases worldwide. Here are some key points about the prevalence of tooth decay:

1. **Children and adolescents:** Tooth decay is very common in children and adolescents. It is estimated that between 60% and 90% of school-age children worldwide have tooth decay.

2. **Adults:** Almost 100% of adults have had cavities at some point in their lives.

3. **Regional variations:** The prevalence of caries can vary significantly between different regions and countries, depending on factors such as access to dental care, diet, fluoride use and public health policies.

4. **Risk factors:** high sugar consumption, lack of access to oral health services and inadequate dental hygiene are important risk factors for the development of cavities.

5. **Socioeconomic impact:** Low-income populations generally have a higher prevalence of caries due to limited access to dental health services and oral care products.

Although tooth decay is preventable, it still represents a significant burden for many people and health systems around the world. Oral health education, access to preventive treatments such as fissure sealing and fluoride use, and the promotion of a healthy diet are key to reducing the prevalence of tooth decay.

Dental caries is a multifactorial disease, as it is infectious, transmissible and sucrose-dependent. It requires the interaction between pathogenic microorganisms and a cariogenic diet, in a host that offers a suitable environment, for a certain period of time. It is closely linked to the introduction of refined carbohydrates into the population's diet, especially sucrose, which is considered the most cariogenic disaccharide and is the most present in the family diet in almost the entire world. It has affected the oral cavity since prehistoric times. The great variation in human susceptibility to caries was and is influenced by cultural and dietary factors at any time in history. The decline in caries disease that has occurred worldwide in recent decades is attributed to the widespread use of fluoride compounds. Therefore, it is possible and should be taken into consideration the use of fluoride, with the aim of promoting oral health (Mondelli *et al.*, 2004; Novais *et al.*, 2004; Bijella *et al.*, 2005; Delbem *et al.*, 2006; De Almeida *et al.*, 2007).

Fluoride has been used in dentistry for many years and its efficiency is essential. There are numerous ways to find fluoride, from fluoridated toothpastes, mouthwashes, chewing gum and even in water supplies, to which fluoride is added in order to obtain its anticariogenic power, which is so important to public health (Schuller & Kalsbeek, 2003; Felix *et al.*, 2004; Hellwig & Lennon, 2004; Ten Cate, 2004; Bijella *et al.*, 2005). However, it has been underused and often misused due to controversies created without scientific evidence.

Despite the important and undeniable advances in oral health, there is still a long way to go. Caries is far from being considered under control, much less on the verge of extinction, even in developed countries. This is also due to the way it is approached by society and the competent bodies (Schuller & Kalsbeek 2003; Ten Cate, 2004).

Fluoride has been shown to be a therapeutic agent that modulates dental caries. Frequent contact between patients and small concentrations of fluoride hinders demineralization and activates remineralization, in addition to inhibiting cariogenic microorganisms. Fluoride ions are administered through different vehicles; they are chemical elements that are incorporated into the crystalline network of the enamel, making them important for maintaining dental health. This statement is based on the possibility that this drug, particularly in the form of sodium fluoride (NaF), can intervene in the dissolution of this biological structure, satisfactorily reducing mineral loss and, consequently, helping to prevent and control dental caries. As a preventive resource, fluoride is a pharmacological alternative used in public health programs, given its significant efficacy and low cost of application (Felix *et al.*, 2004; Ten Cate, 2004; Rouxel *et al.*, 2008).

The diagnosis and treatment of caries have focused and continue to focus on the sequelae of the disease, the caries cavity, focusing on surgical treatment to restore the mineralized tissues of the teeth. Due to the limited benefit of restorative treatment, a reconsideration of conventional procedures is inevitable. Conceptual changes, associated with technological and scientific development, directly influence clinical procedures aimed at promoting oral health, including minimally invasive ultraconservative preparations and the selection of appropriate materials for a holistic approach to the patient. The use of fluoride has been recommended due to low levels of fluoride and in a frequent manner, in which it is possible to reduce enamel demineralization and increase remineralization (Delbem *et al.*, 2006).

This book emerged from a public health specialization project in 2013 and was developed in 2015, after completing my PhD research, in which we analyzed around 900 children and adolescents and were able to evaluate the extremely high amount of cavities, observed by the CPO-D index, a unit of **measurement dental** clinic that evaluates **decayed, missing** and **filled teeth**; and how much this influenced the quality of life of those affected, preventing them from eating, studying, playing sports or even smiling. And so we really resumed the project, as a priority, in 2024. Because tooth decay only increases in proportion to the population. And without a doubt it can be contained worldwide.

As a professor of Public Health at the Amazonas State University (UEA) for 5 years, I was able to evaluate more than 10,000 schoolchildren and their mouths, and as a dental surgeon at the Municipal Health Department (Semsa) in Manaus for over 13 years, I have certainly treated more than 30,000 people of all ages. Tooth decay and its consequences, combined with the lack of interest from the government, have fueled the crucial need for an attitude that can truly change global public health.

This, combined with over 10 years of experience working at the Check UP Hospital in Manaus, Amazonas state, Brazil, specializing in Highly Complex Cardiological and Neurological Surgery since 2012. We provide excellent care to patients at imminent risk of death and save them. However, many of these patients have untreated intraoral chromic lesions that, if left untreated, will reinfect the individuals, often requiring surgical intervention and replacement of their heart valves due to bacterial endocarditis. With all our work, we can reduce our rates to almost zero, by reaffirming assisted dental treatment with medical approval in highly complex cases.

As we are on all fronts, from prevention for children to extremely complex medical care for patients on their deathbeds, trying to save them, and also serving the indigenous community of the Amazon, Easterners, Europeans, North Americans, industries based in the Manaus Free Trade Zone, and even Venezuelan and Haitian refugees, that is, every possible type of patient worldwide, we can witness the entire catastrophic chain caused by the lack of active protocols for preventing cavities, water fluoridation, and a diet based on simple carbohydrates, flour, and derivatives.

In Manaus, the state capital of over 2 million inhabitants, according to the IBGE, the center of the Amazon rainforest, with acidic water, caused by many reasons and also due to organic matter and decomposition of leaves, coming from the Rio Negro and its tributaries, and without water fluoridation, without basic sanitation and with other problems, with an immense extension, even larger than many European countries, for example, without road access in the state capital, only with river and air transport, when we go to the interior this multiplies exponentially. In addition to having high rates of children with autism, which say it is directly influenced by fluoride, according to some articles, however in our state we do not have fluoridation, so this statement does not make sense, being one of the hypotheses for the increase in the prevalence of autism the high amount of mercury in the water due to illegal mining around the Amazon, which should be scientifically investigated.

When a child does not brush their teeth and cavities begin to develop, they can lead to an infection, which is associated with painful symptoms, decreased immunity and cognitive capacity. In most cases, the disease will progress and the possibly infected baby teeth will pass on the cavities to the permanent teeth, which grow at an average age of 6. Since the bacteria is present in the mouths of 98% of the world's population, without proper care, the prognosis will be the worst possible. It is worth remembering that, compared to age groups worldwide, the permanent tooth grows at 6 years of age, in this case the first molar, but in warm environments there is scientific evidence that this tooth grows earlier, at 5 years of age. Parents of all ages and socioeconomic levels do not realize that this tooth is permanent and the child will be mutilated for the rest of their life if they lose it.

Thus, water fluoridation at treatment plants has been mandatory in Brazil since 1974, according to Federal Law No. 6,050/19741, which has not yet been implemented and generates billions of reais in financial and psychological losses, as not having teeth affects a person's life forever. In such a way that they will not be able to eat or bite properly, causing headaches, among several other pathologies.

This work is not just a bibliographic review, it is a compilation of 75 years of true clinical and academic dentistry by two professionals who are fully focused on our science, in all aspects of public health and high-tech dentistry with Invisalign, CT scans, prototyping, dental scanners and everything that is most modern on the market. And it aims to highlight the importance of fluoride for public health, analyzing its various presentations and evaluating its anti-cariogenic power, with the aim of highlighting fluoride as an extremely cheap and effective medicine for reducing the prevalence of tooth decay, while evaluating its pros and cons, thereby encouraging its use in Global Public Health, associating it and defining it as the real vaccine against tooth decay, simple, cheap and available on the market, obviously well administered, with criteria and care. In addition to creating a World Oral Health Campaign in March, called Black March, to highlight the latent need for change throughout the month.

2

FLUORIDE

Fluorine is a chemical element, symbol F, with atomic number 9 (9 protons and 9 electrons), atomic mass 19 u, located in the halogen group (group 17 or VIIA) of the periodic table of elements.

In its biatomic form (F_2) and at STP, it is a pale yellow gas. It is the most electronegative and reactive of all the elements. In its ionized form (F^-) it is extremely dangerous and can cause severe chemical burns if in contact with living tissue.

- At NTP, fluorine is a corrosive, pale yellow gas that is highly oxidizing. It is the most electronegative and most reactive nonmetallic element and forms compounds with virtually all other elements, including the noble gases xenon and radon. Even in the absence of light and at low temperatures, it reacts explosively with hydrogen. Jets of fluorine in the gaseous state attack glass, metals, water, and other substances, which react to form a bright flame. Fluorine is always found in combination in nature and has an affinity for many elements, especially silicon, and cannot be stored in glass containers.

In aqueous solutions of its salts, fluorine is normally present in the form of fluoride ions, F^-. Other forms are fluorine complexes such as $[FeF_4]^-$ or H_2F^+.

Fluorides are compounds in which fluoride ions are bonded to some positively charged chemical residue.

Fluoride is not considered an essential mineral element for humans [1]. Small amounts of fluoride can benefit bone strengthening, but its lack is only a problem in the formulation of artificial diets.

In 1990, Harvard toxicologist Phillis Mullenix showed that fluoride caused IQ to decrease and increased symptoms of attention deficit hyperactivity disorder (ADHD) in rats. Just days before his research was accepted for publication, Mullenix was fired as head of toxicology at the Forsyth Dental Center in Boston. Subsequently, his application for a grant to continue his research on the effects of fluoride on the central nervous system was rejected by the National

Institutes of Health (NIH), when an NIH panel told him that "fluoride has no effects on the central nervous system" (Griffiths 1998).

Fluorine (from the Latin *fluere* = "to flow"), which forms part of the mineral fluorite, CaF_2, was described in 1529 by Georgius Agricola for its use as a flux, used to reduce the melting points of metals or minerals. In 1670 Heinrich Schwanhard observed that it was possible to etch glass when exposed to fluorite that had been treated with acid. Later, Carl Wilhelm Scheele, Humphry Davy, Gay-Lussac, Antoine Lavoisier and Louis Thenard carried out experiments with hydrofluoric acid. Some of these experiments ended in tragedy. Fluorine was discovered in 1771 by Carl Wilhelm Scheele; however, due to its high reactivity, it was not possible to isolate it because, when separated from some compound, it immediately reacted with other substances. Finally, in 1886, it was isolated by the French chemist Henri Moissan.

The first commercial production of fluorine was for the atomic bomb of the Manhattan Project, to obtain uranium hexafluoride, UF_6, used for the separation of uranium isotopes.

The first studies on fluoride ingestion in humans were conducted in Nazi concentration camps with the aim of calming the prisoners, who ingested the ion from water with up to 1500 ppm of fluoride. The result generated a kind of stupor; the prisoners performed their tasks better without questioning them. With the same objective, fluoride is added to some psychiatric medications today. More than 60 widely used tranquilizers contain fluoride, such as Diazepam, Valium and Rohypnol, from Roche, linked to the former IG Farben, a chemical company that worked in the service of Nazi Germany (Source: http://www.theforbiddenknowledge.com/hardtruth/fluoridation.htm). Fluoride was also used as a rat poison.

Fluorine is the most abundant halogen in the Earth's crust, with a concentration of 950 ppm. In seawater it is found in a proportion of approximately 1.3 ppm. The most important minerals in which it is present are fluorite, CaF_2, fluorapatite, $Ca_5(PO_4)_3F$ and cryolite, Na_3AlF_6.

It is obtained by the electrolysis of a mixture of HF and KF. In the process, the oxidation of fluorides occurs at the anode:

$$2F^- - 2e^- \rightarrow F_2$$

Hydrogen is discharged at the cathode, and it is necessary to prevent the two gases obtained from coming into contact to avoid the risk of explosion.

Fluoride is also an effluent byproduct of aluminum production.

- Numerous organic compounds are used in which hydrogen atoms have been formally replaced by fluorine atoms. There are different ways of obtaining them, one of the most important being through substitution reactions of other halogens:

$$CHCl_3 + 2HF \rightarrow CHClF_2 + 2HCl$$

- CFCs have been used in a wide variety of applications, such as refrigerants, propellants, foaming agents, insulators, etc. However, as they contributed to the destruction of the ozone layer, they were replaced by other chemical compounds, such as HCFs. HCFCs are also used as replacements for CFCs, but they also destroy the ozone layer in the long term.

- Polytetrafluoroethylene (PTFE) is a polymer called Teflon, with high chemical resistance and a low coefficient of friction.

- Hydrofluoric acid is an aqueous solution of hydrogen fluoride. It is a weak acid, but much more dangerous than strong acids such as hydrochloric acid. HF acid is used to etch glass and to remove silica (sand) from special steels.

- Uranium hexafluoride, UF_6, is a room temperature gas used to separate uranium isotopes.

- Fluorine forms compounds with other halogens, in which case the oxidation state is -1, for example, IF_7, BrF_5, BrF_3, and ClF.

- Natural cryolite, Na_3AlF_6, is a mineral containing fluorides. It was mined in Greenland, but is now practically exhausted. Fortunately, it can be obtained synthetically and used to obtain aluminum by electrolysis.

Fluoride is present in mammals in the form of fluorides. Although its necessary consumption has not been proven (WHO, 2002, Guidelines for Water Quality), it is allegedly a very reactive and toxic substance. It accumulates in bones and teeth, making them less resistant. Therefore, its addition to water, salt and milk by chemists, technicians and engineers is unnecessary.

Fluoride is usually added to toothpastes at levels of around 1000ppm to 1500ppm, which should not be swallowed. It is also strictly prohibited for children under 6 years of age.

Is also added to water in small quantities (0.6 ppm - 1.0 ppm) because it is very toxic. The World Health Organization (WHO) considers fluoride to be a medicine, but approves its addition to water, milk or salt as an effective way to combat tooth decay, although this has never been proven.

Fluoridation was implemented in Brazil during the government of former President Ernesto Geisel. However, the laws on fluoridation of public water were recently challenged by politicians and other professionals opposed to the mass treatment of the population, in the Senate and Chamber of Deputies, which considered it unethical, according to their values, while they were celebrated by medical organizations and scientific communities.

Thus, ethical questions have been raised regarding this mass medication without a prescription. And that people with some degree of autism are even more harmed by mandatory fluoridation, including of food, since this is a depressant of the central nervous system.

The WHO also recommends that research be carried out into sources of fluoride other than water, to determine whether people are already exposed to unnecessary levels of the element in the air and food. Unfortunately, this practice is rarely practiced in Brazil. It is the job of dentists, public authorities and scientists to ensure that excessive use of the substance is punishable by severe penalties for those who use it (industry, water treatment plant technicians, etc.), and that the correct limits are used in order to reduce tooth decay with minimal side effects, as well as to ensure treatment for victims of unsightly fluorosis (relatively rare).

It is worth remembering that some waters are naturally fluoridated. Bottled mineral waters follow fluoridation laws. Therefore, fluoridation is not as efficient and necessary as advertised.

Fluoride, which comes from artificial fluoridation, is absorbed in excessive quantities by the human body and is difficult to excrete. Most of it is deposited in the solid parts of the mammalian organism, the bone tissue, while a small portion travels to the teeth. Organic fluorides may be essential nutrients, but this possibility has not yet been proven, although a normal human being has an average of 500 ppm/F in the bones of the body.

Fluoride poisoning is known as dental fluorosis, and manifests itself as brittle and discolored teeth. It usually occurs when children consume large amounts of fluoridated water, both unnatural and naturally added, as they are in the process of growth and bone formation, and in foods processed with this water. Therefore, it is important for children to be supplemented with calcium and iodine so that they do not suffer from poor mineralization with defective Fluorite crystals (CaF2) and thyroid problems. The list of effects can be summarized as follows, for the consumption of fluoride compounds:

- 6.0 mg /day — harmful effects, presence of bone and neurological problems in some children and mild, moderate and severe fluorosis with serious aesthetic impairment. Many people can tolerate this portion well.

- 10.0 mg /day to 20 mg/day — toxic amount. Some people may experience gastric problems due to the formation of HF in the stomach. This amount can lead to bone diseases such as skeletal fluorosis, arthritis, and stress fractures, associated with learning disabilities in infants. It corresponds to problems reported by UNICEF in Indian and Chinese communities. It is linked to problems reported by people living near ceramic and fertilizer factories and consumers of unsafe water in the Brazilian Northeast. Water with more than 1.5 ppm should be treated with adsorption, flocculation, distillation, or reverse osmosis.

- 200 mg — deaths due to poisoning in children have been reported at this dosage. It causes severe gastric discomfort due to the formation of hydrofluoric acid (HF) in the stomach and consequent injury to the gastric mucosa.

- 500 mg – 2g — 500 mg in a single dose can cause cardiac arrest and death in children, and doses of 2g or more of sodium fluoride can kill an adult. Gastric lavage and consumption of lime water Ca(OH)2, magnesium hydroxide, or milk can reduce the body's absorption of the substance. It is essential that the patient be taken to a hospital for treatment.

Fluoride and HF must be handled with great care, and any contact with the skin or eyes must be avoided. They must also not be stored in glass containers, as they corrode.

Both fluoride and fluoride ions are highly toxic. Fluoride has a characteristic pungent odor and is detectable at concentrations as low as 0.02 ppm, below the recommended exposure limits.

Fluoride is more toxic than lead, and its level in drinking water should not exceed 0.4 parts per million (ppm). The fluoride level in drinking water is usually 1.5 ppm.

In Sicily, a relationship was found between regions with high concentrations of fluoride in the water and the occurrence of serious dental diseases.

The FDA considers fluoride to be an unapproved drug, for which there is no evidence of its safety or effectiveness.

- Analytical methods

According to the Standards Methods for Water and Wastewater, 22nd edition, the most commonly used methods for determining fluoride are by colorimetry, via SPADNS, and by selective ion. As explained previously, it is very important to control fluoride levels, both in drinking water and in effluents. According to ordinance 2914 of 12/12/2011 of the Ministry of Health, the maximum permitted level for fluoride in drinking water is 1.5 mg /L, as excess fluoride can be harmful.

- What is fluoride?

Fluoride is a naturally occurring mineral found throughout the Earth's crust and is widely distributed in nature. Some foods and water supplies contain fluoride.

Fluoride is commonly added to drinking water to help reduce cavities. In the 1930s, researchers found that people who grew up drinking naturally fluoridated water had up to two-thirds fewer cavities than people living in areas without fluoridated water. Studies since then have repeatedly shown that when fluoride is added to a community's water supply, tooth decay decreases. The American Dental Association, the World Health Organization, and the American Medical Association, among many other organizations, have endorsed the use of fluoride in water supplies because of its effect on tooth decay.

- How does fluoride work?

Fluoride helps prevent cavities in two different ways:
- Fluoride concentrates in the growing bones and developing teeth of children, helping to harden the enamel of baby and adult teeth before they erupt.

- Fluoride helps harden the enamel of permanent teeth that have already emerged.
- Fluoride works during the demineralization and remineralization processes that naturally occur in your mouth.
- After eating, your saliva contains acids that cause demineralization, the dissolution of calcium and phosphorus beneath the tooth surface.
- At other times, when your saliva is less acidic, it does just the opposite, replacing the calcium and phosphorus that keep your teeth hard. This process is called remineralization. When fluoride is present during remineralization, the deposited minerals are harder than they would otherwise be, helping to strengthen your teeth and prevent dissolution during the next phase of demineralization.

- How do I know if I'm getting enough fluoride?

If your drinking water is fluoridated, then regular brushing with a fluoride toothpaste is considered sufficient for adults and children with healthy teeth and a low risk of tooth decay.

If your community water is not fluoridated and does not have enough natural fluoride (one part per million is considered ideal), then your dentist or pediatrician may prescribe fluoride supplements for your children to take daily. Your dentist or pediatrician can tell you how much fluoride is right for your family, so be sure to ask for their advice.

If your water comes from a public water supply, you can find out if it contains fluoride by calling your local water company. If your water comes from a private well, you can have it tested by an independent environmental testing company that provides water testing services.

3

WHAT IS A VACCINE?

A **vaccine** is a biological preparation that provides active acquired immunity to a particular infectious disease. Vaccines contain agents that resemble a disease-causing microorganism and are often made from attenuated or killed forms of the microorganism, its toxins, or one of its surface proteins.

3.1 How Vaccines Work

1. **Stimulation of the Immune System:** When a vaccine is administered, it stimulates the immune system to recognize the agent as a threat, destroy it, and "remember" it so that the body can quickly recognize and destroy the microorganism when exposed to it in the future.

2. **Active Immunity:** Vaccines induce an active immune response without causing disease, preparing the body to defend itself against future infections. This helps prevent disease or reduce its severity.

3. **Types of Vaccines:**

- **Inactivated or Killed Vaccines:** Made from viruses or bacteria that have been killed or inactivated so that they cannot cause disease.

- **Live Attenuated Vaccines:** contain a weakened form of the virus or bacteria that is still capable of inducing an immune response without causing disease.

- **Subunit, Recombinant, Polysaccharide and Conjugate Vaccines:** use specific parts of the pathogen, such as proteins or sugars, to stimulate an immune response.

- **Toxoid vaccines:** Made from toxins (harmful chemicals) produced by bacteria. The toxins are inactivated so they cannot cause disease.

- **RNA vaccines:** These contain a piece of messenger RNA (mRNA) that encodes a protein from the pathogen, allowing the body's cells to produce that protein and trigger an immune response.

3.2 Benefits of Vaccines

- **Disease Prevention:** Vaccines are one of the most effective tools for preventing infectious diseases and have contributed to the eradication or control of diseases such as smallpox, polio, measles and tetanus.
- **Herd Immunity:** When a high percentage of the population is vaccinated, the spread of infectious diseases is reduced, providing protection also for those who cannot be vaccinated, such as people with certain health conditions.
- **Reduction of Morbidity and Mortality:** Vaccines significantly reduce the morbidity (severity of disease) and mortality (death rate) associated with many infectious diseases.

Vaccines are an essential component of public health and continue to be an area of intense research and innovation, especially in responding to new infectious threats.

3.3 The ideal vaccine

The effectiveness of a vaccine is assessed by how well it protects against a specific disease. There are two important concepts related to this.

Efficacy: This refers to a vaccine's ability to prevent disease in a controlled setting, such as clinical trials. For example, if a vaccine is 90% effective, it means that 90 out of every 100 people vaccinated will be protected from the disease. However, 10 of those 100 people who receive the vaccine may still get sick.

Effectiveness: This represents how the vaccine works in the general population, under real-world conditions. In other words, it takes into account factors such as people's genetic variability, different environments and exposures. Effectiveness can be different from efficacy, as it takes the broader scenario into account.

Here are some updated data on the effectiveness of some Covid-19 vaccines in Brazil:

AstraZeneca:
Overall efficacy: 76% in preventing symptomatic disease (after 15 days or more after 2nd dose).

Protection against the delta variant: 92% in preventing hospitalizations.

Prevention of serious illness: 100%.

Prevention of hospitalizations: 92%.

Infection prevention: 69% to 92% (after 2 doses).

CoronaVac (Butantan Institute):

Overall effectiveness: 50.38%.

Protection against the delta variant: data not yet available to the same extent as for other vaccines.

Please note that these numbers may change based on new research and variants of the virus. Full vaccination is essential for maximum protection.

The ideal vaccine, according to the WHO, must have some specific characteristics to be considered ideal in the Brazilian context:

1. High efficacy: the vaccine must provide protection against severe and moderate disease.

2. Low production cost: This is important to make immunization affordable.

3. Single dose: Ideally, the vaccine would be administered as a single dose, although this may not be possible.

4. Thermostability: the vaccine must be stable at temperatures between 2°C and 8°C, as the country's cold chain offers this temperature range.

3.4 Would fluoride as a vaccine be possible?

If a vaccine is around 50% to 75% efficient depending on factors related to the immunity of each patient, it is like the flu vaccine, which does not cause the complete disappearance of the disease so that the person does not need to take it again, which can affect the patient, and needs to be readministered annually with the insertion of new strains.

Using the correct administration of fluoride with glass ionomer cement sealant annually, and obviously associated with DAILY measures, which are: the use of dental floss, proper tooth brushing and the use of fluoride mouthwash before going to bed, even with water fluoridation carried out in a controlled manner, it is almost impossible for a person to be affected by cavities.

If we remove so many associated variables and perform sealant placement on schoolchildren aged 5 to 6, repeating it annually, our clinical practice leads us to believe that cavities will be practically negative. This will enable full health, after all, health starts in the mouth and cavities need to be reviewed as a universal disease that needs to be controlled.

Therefore, the proposal of this book is as a protocol for treating all patients in this age group and reassessing them in previous years, as a vaccination measure, as it is an advancing disease and one of the most prevalent worldwide.

The spatulated glass ionomer cement in a pasty/plastic phase is applied in a thin layer to the area of dental scars and fissures, releasing fluoride in the areas of occlusion and masticatory contact, which are the areas most likely to be affected by cavities. This will drastically reduce the incidence of cavities and may even eliminate them if the DAILY measures are carried out satisfactorily.

3.5 Fluoride as a vaccine against tooth decay in the world

It is known that public health in the world is guided by generally restorative measures and with extremely expensive treatments throughout the world, where prevention should be carried out with protective measures, based on education and the reduction of diseases with great impact and with great destructive power on general health, especially those that generate high costs for human health and for governments around the world, with a high prevalence x costs x disability ratio, such as: diabetes, hypertension, cardiovascular diseases and tooth decay.

Dental caries is a universal disease with high treatment costs and worsening quality of life, but with very low prevention costs, linked to educational measures and the "anti-cavity vaccine", carried out through a continuous protocol before the age of 5, an important phase that precedes the eruption or birth of the first permanent tooth. And with recurring reassessments every 6 months. Care should also be taken with periodontal or gum disease.

3.6 Anti-cavity protocol and its vaccine

Performed based on a protocol before the age of 2 with the emergence of all baby molars and mainly after the age of 5, an important phase that precedes the eruption or emergence of the first permanent tooth.

Obviously, the child needs to be monitored from birth with biannual visits to the dentist, and parents should be taught how to brush their teeth after meals and the necessary care to prevent cavities from spreading.

Conventionalizing this methodology in a proportionally better way than many injectable vaccine protocols, in which the patient can still be affected by the disease, such as the flu vaccine, which obviously has value for the health of an entire population, but this prevention should also be carried out with low financial cost and with great potential for resolution.

Where the sealant with spatulated restorative glass ionomer cement is applied directly to the dental grooves of newly erupted teeth, there is a high prevalence of caries.

Our 55 years of clinical and academic experience (Dr. João Batista) and 17 years (Dr. Thiago Noronha) working in Dentistry with thousands of patients, from the highest purchasing power, with million-dollar planes, to the poorest, in some cases refugees from other countries, such as Venezuela, Haiti, or those who live in communities in the Amazon, with access to the capital Manaus only by a 5- day boat trip. Or even patients from the Middle East, Europe, Asia and the United States, because we are in Manaus, in the Manaus Free Trade Zone, a manufacturing city with multinational companies (Samsung, Honda and Sony from the East, Bic and Essilor, which are European, Procter and Gamble, which is North American, and others), gives us immense global experience and experience.

Thus, all this accumulated experience of more than 70 years with patients from literally all over the world makes us believe that tooth decay is universal, prevalent in all age groups and socioeconomic groups, causing harm to all races, creeds and all social classes.

Often increased by the sugar epidemic in the world, by the food industry, which will be the food for the bacteria *Streptococcus mutans* to develop and destroy the dental structure.

Remembering that in rich countries access to a professional dentist is difficult because it is also expensive, and this increases the rate of tooth decay, and simple cavities become bigger problems with missing teeth and creating occlusal problems, headaches and even generalized infections.

It is essential that governments worldwide take a strong stance, as this is the best possible method of preventing tooth decay. Quick, simple and effective.

Often masked by possible effects of fluoride on syndromes, which is not fully scientifically proven, remembering that all proposed treatment is carried out topically and without direct ingestion of the fluoride itself, eliminating any possible questions about the subject.

This article has already been attempted to be published, but it was not possible because it is a "very simple" method and would not bring great financial gain to large companies.

Being forgotten and not evaluated in a concrete and solid way as the real transforming agent of this disease so common in the four corners of the world, which could indeed be avoided.

And I ask you, reader, to do a self-analysis, that is, to assess how many cavities or missing teeth you have had. If the answer is no, I ask you to also evaluate the amount of dental calculus or tartar you have, as I am almost certain that you have already been affected by one of these oral pathologies, demonstrating once again the importance of this issue for the entire world, in which any measure will have a positive impact not only on individuals like you and me, but on the entire world. After all, health education transforms lives.

3.7 Fluoride as a major modifier of quality of life and global health

Our co-author, Dr. João Batista Filgueiras de Noronha, graduated in Dentistry since 1970, in 2025 will complete 55 years of daily dental activity, having clinical activity in a private practice and being a retired professor with more than 35 years of teaching at the Federal University of Amazonas and another 10 years at the State University of Amazonas.

Along with the experience of the author, a public health specialist, master and PhD in dental clinics, as well as a professor and dentist in a high-end private clinic, in a hospital and also in public service, with 17 years of experience. We have always supported the hypothesis that fluoride changes people's quality of life, while reducing "mutilation" due to tooth extraction and its complications after its removal, in which the tooth is seen as an organ of the human body that is being radically removed, most likely caused by tooth decay in 95% of cases. And in these 55 years of daily dentistry, treating patients from all social classes, from the rich to the middle class and from the poor to the very poor and refugees, treated in educational institutions because it is the last call for the cry of pain, in which the pain caused by the tooth does cause death and is notoriously one of the 3 most profound pains that a human being can have.

Care which is often provided to patients who live in the interior of Amazonas, completely remotely, who sometimes need 5 days to arrive by boat at the place of care (Noronha, Moneiro, 2024)

We have seen in recent years that the only agent for transforming oral health is fluoride in its various forms, the most effective being water fluoridation combined with sealing the occlusal surface (where we eat) with type R glass ionomer cement.

A simple, effective and inexpensive action that should be carried out at the age of 6 when the first permanent upper and lower molars erupt or "grow".

Sense obviously replaced every 6 months, when this product falls out, which attaches to the tooth in an extremely simple way and with fantastic effectiveness.

In almost 55 years of experience, this has undoubtedly been the best way to reduce the incidence of cavities. Leading to the long-awaited zero cavities rate, repeatedly, and it is incredible in the sense that the child will become an adult without cavities.

In a completely clinical manner, in the day-to-day practice of dentistry in its essence, reviewing patients and following them for years and decades in our clinical practice. Even in patients with Down Syndrome or Autism, we eliminate caries activity, without any distorted academic bias, due to the simple and mere issue of economic power.

This proposal has been made to politicians many times, but has never been taken into consideration because it is so simple, incredibly effective and cheap. Obviously, it has been treated this way by ulterior motives.

This measure would drastically reduce problems in the oral cavity, reducing costs for public health, dental treatments and general medical care. Medical professionals are often unaware of the dangers of oral infections because they are not familiar with the oral cavity. In many medical and other medical science courses, they are not taught the basics to know how to recommend treatment by the dentist. This means that patients do not go to the dentist, feeling a lot of pain or often even dying from bacterial endocarditis or sepsis in a hospital, with indefinite autopsy reports in some cases.

Like the notorious case of the soccer player, the star Ronaldo Fenômeno, Ronaldo Nazário, winner of two World Cups for Brazil, had an infection in his mouth that reduced his potential for technical and athletic performance. And when he went to the Cruzeiro team of the State of Minas Gerais, in Brazil, at the age of 16, the infection was discovered and treated, after which he became a great player, reaching his maximum potential and becoming one of the greatest soccer players in the world. In other words, pain and infection do not combine with elite physical performance or with intellectual or cognitive activities.

The cascade effect could be mitigated by a simple measure, such as glass ionomer cement, a restorative type used in children, which seals the surface and also releases fluoride continuously, making the tooth "stronger" and less prone to cavities. Among other possibilities, such as water fluoridation.

The percentage of children in the world who are mature enough to brush their teeth at 5 or 6 years old, who understand that foods with sugar will destroy their mouth with cavities if they do not brush with fluoride, is tiny. So this quick sealant procedure will reflect on their entire life, causing prevention.

This information is of a generalist and universal nature, obviously more relevant to the general dental profession, specifically for public health as a whole, but also for the entire world population who will indeed benefit from something for years, therefore our unwavering recommendation is to apply this product to all children in the world and reapplication when necessary, due to lack of it on the occlusal or chewing surface, until at least the person can brush their teeth truly effectively.

Obviously this prevents it, but flossing and possibly rinsing your mouth with fluoride before going to bed without ingesting it will indeed lead this patient to the much dreamed of and almost utopian "zero cavities".

4

LITERATURE REVIEW

The Brazilian National Oral Health Policy has as its guiding principles: actions to promote and protect health, including water fluoridation, health education, supervised oral hygiene, topical fluoride applications and recovery and rehabilitation of oral health (Brazil, 2009).

Oral health promotion is part of a broad concept of health that transcends dentistry, uniting oral health with other collective health practices. Thus, it means the creation of healthy public policies, the development of strategies aimed at the entire community, such as policies that can create opportunities for access to treated water, encouraging water fluoridation, the use of fluoridated toothpaste and ensuring the availability of appropriate basic dental care. Health promotion actions also include working with approaches to simultaneous risk or protective factors, both for oral cavity diseases and for other conditions (diabetes, hypertension, obesity, trauma and cancer), such as: healthy eating policies to reduce sugar consumption, community approaches to increase the person's own care with body and oral hygiene, policies to eliminate smoking and reduce accidents (Brazil, 1998; Brazil, 2004).

When identifying the main groups of actions for health promotion, protection and recovery, it is necessary to analyze and understand the characteristics of the epidemiological profile of the population, not only in terms of diseases with greater prevalence, but also the socioeconomic conditions of the community, their habits, lifestyles and their health needs, including by extension the infrastructure of available services (Brazil, 2004).

The dental practice model in Brazil was designed and targeted at children aged 6 to 12, pregnant women and babies, prioritizing individual and curative care. Public actions offered to the adult population are generally focused on emergency restorative care and have not undergone significant changes since the implementation of the Unified Health System (SUS) in 1990. As a consequence of this type of service offered to the economically active population, there has been a worsening of oral health conditions and, consequently, an increase in the prevalence of pain of odontogenic origin. This has a direct impact on absenteeism, as workers are unable to perform their activities, which will cause a decrease in production and profits, which goes against the economic policy of any company, whether public or private (Lacerda *et al.*, 2008).

The prevalence of painful episodes originating from the oral cavity has been high and increasing in recent times. In the recent national survey on oral health conditions, it was observed that 33.7% of the population between 15 and 74 years of age reported having felt pain in the six months prior to the survey, and of these, approximately 9% stated having felt intense pain. Toothache is experienced as a difficulty faced by populations and individuals who do not find appropriate means for oral health care in health services (Lacerda *et al.*, 2008).

Midorikawa (2000) reports that approximately 25% of absenteeism due to non-occupational diseases is directly related to oral conditions. Toothache is the third most common cause of absence from work, behind only stomachache and headache. Poor attendance at work due to health reasons, in addition to directly interfering with productivity, can, for reasons related to pain and lack of concentration, lead to depression, anxiety and irritability, increasing the risk of technical errors, interpersonal conflicts and work accidents.

Dental caries can be defined as a process of dissolution of enamel or dentin, caused by bacterial action on the tooth surface and mediated by a physical-chemical flow of ions dissolved in water. It is a direct product of the continuous variation of the pH of the oral cavity, being the result of successive cycles of demineralization and remineralization (DES x RE) of minerals present in saliva, such as calcium and phosphate, on the tooth surface, and the loss of the "DES X RE" balance occurs when the pH falls below 5.5 or 4.5 in the presence of fluoride (Soares & Valença, 2003).

Dental caries is caused by the accumulation of bacteria on the teeth and frequent exposure to fermentable sugars. Thus, when sugar is ingested, the bacteria present in dental plaque (biofilm) produce acids that demineralize (dissolve) the mineral structure of the teeth while the pH remains low (<6.7 for dentin and <5.5 for enamel). After a certain period of exposure to sugar, the pH rises to values above the critical ones for enamel-dentin and saliva tends to replace the dissolved minerals, through a phenomenon called remineralization (Brasil, 2009; Kwon *et al.*, 2010).

The minerals of the enamel-dentin structure are dissolved by acids and the mineral fluorapatite (FA) is less soluble than hydroxyapatite (HA). In the past, it was believed that, once incorporated into the tooth structure, FA would make the tooth less soluble to the acids produced in the dental biofilm (plaque).

However, the concentration of F found in the enamel formed upon exposure to F does not reach 10% FA, a value that does not significantly reduce the solubility of the tooth to acids of bacterial origin. Thus, F incorporated systemically into the dental mineral has a very limited effect on caries control (Brasil, 2009).

However, since FA is a less soluble mineral, it has a greater tendency to precipitate in enamel and dentin than HA during demineralization and remineralization. Thus, even if the drop in pH generated in the dental biofilm by exposure to carbohydrates favors the dissolution of HA, if there is fluoride ion present in the oral environment (dental biofilm fluid, saliva), FA will still have a tendency to precipitate. Consequently, in a certain pH range, there will be dissolution of HA and, concomitantly, precipitation of FA, counterbalancing the net mineral loss of the dental structure and, consequently, delaying the development of caries lesions. Thus, 5.5 should be considered the critical pH for the enamel of an individual or population not exposed daily to any of the forms of fluorides. When exposed to F, the critical pH drops to 4.5 and, thus, between this value and 5.5, at the same time that the tooth loses minerals in the form of HA, a certain amount of dissolved calcium and phosphate ions returns to the tooth in the form of FA (Brazil, 2009).

The net result of this physical-chemical phenomenon caused by the simple presence of F in the medium is a reduction in the demineralization of enamel-dentin. Additionally, when the pH of the biofilm returns to neutrality, the F present in the medium activates the remineralizing capacity of saliva and the enamel-dentin has a greater repair of the lost minerals than it would have in the absence of F, that is, there is a potentialization of the remineralizing effect of saliva. Although it may seem unimportant, the constant presence of F in the oral cavity to interact in these physical-chemical events of de- and remineralization that occur daily on the tooth surface, ensuring the saturation of the environment with the ions that make up fluorapatite, is the main mechanism of its action in preventing caries (Brasil, 2009).

Fluoride is used to prevent the appearance of carious lesions, however, fluoride compounds should always be considered as an adjuvant, which, combined with good brushing and a correct diet, will contribute immensely to improving oral health. However, if there are good hygiene and dietary habits, even if not exposed to fluoride, the disease will not develop. This fact highlights the great importance of a good brushing technique for maintaining oral health. In Brazil, fluoridated toothpastes began to be sold on a population scale in 1989. Currently, Brazil is the third country in per capita consumption. of toothpastes, behind only the United States and Japan (Fjerskov *et al.*, 1994; Cury *et al.*, 2004).

Remineralization of dental structures and even the possibility of inhibiting the cytoplasmic metabolism of bacteria involved with dental plaque. In the form of calcium fluoride, this ion becomes an important biological reservoir stored on the enamel surface, a strategy adopted clinically to ensure its topical effect, as long as the prescribed administration is maintained (Felix *et al.*, 2004).

Frequent and repeated use of low concentrations of fluoride promotes salivary levels of fluoride, which is the best way to prevent caries. Levels of 1 to 10 ppm of fluoride reduce enamel solubility and increase remineralization, which facilitates the precipitation of minerals on the enamel surface (Bijella *et al.*, 2005).

The minimum condition for commercial products to have anti-caries potential is the presence of a significant concentration of soluble fluoride in their composition. For example, with the use of a 0.025% solution of neutral sodium fluoride prescribed for daily mouthwash for 30 seconds, an optimal level of protection can be achieved, with an acceptable intake of low levels of fluoride (Felix *et al.*, 2004).

It is important to emphasize that the different administration vehicles for this ion should be considered as essential pharmacological agents for the prevention of dental caries, which does not mean that they can replace the benefits provided by mechanical therapy and the antiplaque activity of antiseptics (Felix *et al.*, 2004).

4.1 Types of fluoride products

4.1.1 Fluoride Mouthwashes

Chemical agents used as antiseptics in the oral cavity date back to 1865, when phenolic agents with essential oils were used as mouthwashes. Currently, there are numerous types of mouthwashes on the market, such as: Listerine, which is a combination of phenol, essential oils, thymol, menthol and menthyl salicylate, mixed in a hydroalcoholic vehicle, used to reduce and control bacterial plaque. Other products, such as Cepacol, which have cetylpyridinium chloride (CCP) as a basic concentrate, also have an antiplaque effect. Preparations based on iodine and chlorine are often used by clinicians as irrigants. They are active against microorganisms and can reduce subgingival plaque (Oliveira, 1996).

Fluoride mouthwashes are solutions that help clean the oral cavity. Their effectiveness depends on continuous use, when a 0.2% sodium fluoride solution, for example, is used. They are only indicated for children aged 6 and over and do not require prior prophylaxis (Chedid, 1999).

Fluoride mouthwashes work by ensuring maximum topical exposure while minimizing the risk of dental fluorosis, since little fluoride is ingested. It is important to use this method at different times of the day to maximize total effectiveness. These substances are not recommended for children under 6 years of age and are indicated for preventing cavities in patients at high risk of cavities. They are used by swishing 10 ml of the solution in the mouth and keeping it in the mouth for one minute (Rouxel *et al.*, 2008).

The application of fluoride in the form of mouthwashes is often associated with antiseptic substances, including cetylpyridinium chloride, triclosan gantrez or chlorhexidine digluconate (Félix *et al.*, 2004).

The use of mouthwash with sodium fluoride (NaF) solution shows positive results in the prevention of dental caries. The recommended solutions for the technique are 0.05% sodium fluoride (227 ppm fluoride) for daily mouthwash and 0.2% (909 ppm fluoride) for weekly mouthwash. An advantageous method has been identified in reducing the incidence of dental caries, strengthening the enamel's resistance capacity (remineralizing and cariostatic action) and enzymatic inhibition of plaque bacteria (Amarante, 1983; Rouxel *et al.*, 2008).

The method allows for continued application and practice of preventive education, and is therefore comprehensive and selective, in addition to having a low cost, which is why it is often chosen as a form of prevention in Public Health. Mouthwashes are indicated as a universal coverage action mainly for municipalities that do not have a fluoridation service for public water supplies and are justified by the prevalence of cavities in the target population. It is also easy and safe to apply, but should be recommended after professional evaluation of its real need, and are not indicated for children under 6 years of age (Amarante, 1983; Rouxel *et al.*, 2008).

Some precautions should be taken regarding fluorosis when using daily mouthwashes, because although the fluoride concentration is low, constant ingestion of the product may pose some risk, especially if used in children under 6 years of age, since they do not have control over their reflexes. Using weekly mouthwashes is safe and does not pose a risk regarding the occurrence of fluorosis. However, ingesting the mouthwash solution daily or weekly may pose some problem regarding acute poisoning, if more than the probably toxic dose, which is 5 mgF/kg, is ingested. In this case, gastrointestinal problems (nausea, vomiting), cardiovascular problems (hypotension) and neurological problems (paresthesia) may occur. All care regarding lethality must be taken when handling the products used (salts, sachets, concentrated solutions) to prepare the solutions, which, in addition to the labeling, must be kept out of the reach of children. In case of accident, administer oral calcium, if necessary induce vomiting with emetics and proceed to hospitalization for control (Frazão *et al.,* 2004; Nunes *et al.,* 2004).

4.1.2 Topical fluoride

Since the 1980s, Brazil has included fluoride gel in some school programs as a preventive agent, with its application through trays. However, due to technical issues, such as the non-distribution of the necessary material, lack of professional support and long-term monitoring, its effectiveness has been questioned. After the 1980s, intensive fluoride therapy was implemented in several municipalities, in which, in addition to health education activities, fluoride gel was used through brushing and fluoride mouthwashes in intensive and maintenance sessions (Cangassu & Costa, 2001).

The products used for applications by dentists are gels and varnishes (there is also a mousse presentation). Fluorinated gels contain 0,9 a1.23% fluoride (9.000 a12,300 ppm F). Varnishes contain 22,600 ppm F. These are products with a high concentration of fluoride and must be handled by qualified professionals, since their use is indicated in intensive fluoride therapy procedures, recommended for individuals at medium and high risk of caries (Barros *et al.,* 2008).

Topical application of professional fluoride is an alternative way to compensate for the patient's lack of self-use of fluoride or lack of preventive measures, and is highly recommended for individuals with greater disease activity (Barros *et al.,* 2008).

There is evidence that the effectiveness of acidulated phosphate fluoride ranges from 20-30% to 30-50% in reducing the prevalence of caries. However, its indiscriminate use, especially by young people, can lead to toxicity that should be avoided (Barros *et al.,* 2008).

Situations in which fluoride gel is used for mass application, indiscriminately, generally once a semester and without prior prophylaxis, should occur when individuals are not exposed to fluoride through other vehicles, or this exposure is minimal, or in cases with a very high prevalence of caries. In these cases, the individual condition is practically not taken into account in defining the strategy (Cangassu & Costa, 2001).

Dentists apply fluoride products in dental clinics to prevent tooth decay. There are several forms of topical fluoride application, such as gel, varnish, and foam. The most common is gel, which contains acidulated phosphate fluoride (APF), which contains 1.23% or 12,300 parts per million (ppm) of fluoride ion and 2% sodium fluoride (NaF), consisting of 0.90% or 9,050 ppm of fluoride ion. Fluoride varnishes usually contain 5% NaF, which is equivalent to 2.26% or 22,600 ppm of fluoride ion. In 1990, fluoride foam was introduced into dental practice. These foams are also indicated for dentin hypersensitivity with exposure of root surfaces or as cavity varnish by the FDA (US Food and Drug Administration), and evidence indicates their effectiveness in preventing cavities (American Dental Association Council On Scientific Affairs, 2006; Barros *et al.*, 2008).

Clinical recommendations for topical fluoride are analyzed and predefined by age and also by the risk of caries. Children aged six years or younger, without risk of caries, may not receive additional benefit from topical application, since fluoridated water and fluoridated toothpaste can provide adequate prevention of caries. Patients with moderate risk need to apply fluoride varnish at six-month intervals, while the application of gel is contraindicated because it contains more fluoride than varnish, therefore it is easier to swallow and also takes less time and discomfort, especially in preschool children. Patients with high risk of caries should have an interval between fluoride varnish applications of between three and six months (Cury *et al.*, 2007).

Patients with low risk of caries aged 6 to 18 years may also not be effective when fluoride is applied, for the same reason as above, which relates to the fact that they already receive fluoride from fluoridated water and fluoridated toothpaste. In cases of moderate risk, fluoride gel or fluoride should be applied every 6 months. Patients with high risk of caries need to be applied every 3 to 6 months, with applications every 3 months being more effective. For people over 18 years of age, the recommendation is identical to that presented. For all ages, fluoride should be applied for 4 minutes, since a duration of only 1 minute is not supported (Cury *et al.*, 2007).

The use of topical fluoride is stratified and recommended based on age and risk of caries, indicating the periodic use of topical fluoride for children and adults, who have a moderate to high risk of developing caries. In this way, the dentist, knowing the patient's health history and vulnerability to developing an oral disease, is in the best position to perform the correct treatment for each patient. Obviously, this choice must have the consensus of the professional and the patient's preferences (Cury *et al.*, 2007).

However, when there is a low prevalence of caries and high exposure to fluoride, the indiscriminate application of fluoride gel is no longer recommended. However, its use remains valid, as long as it is restricted to individuals who actually need it. It can be applied in a clinical setting or in collective spaces. There are several techniques described for each setting, among which we highlight the cotton swab, gauze, tray and toothbrush techniques. The purpose is always the same, the application of fluoride gel, and any technique, to be effective, must be performed appropriately, respecting the steps inherent to each one (Cury *et al.*, 2007). Since the toothbrush technique is the most commonly used in collective actions, it is appropriate to describe it in general terms.

Fluoride Gel Application Technique with a Toothbrush: A small amount of gel, equivalent to a small pea (less than 0.5 g), should be placed in the center of the active tip of a toothbrush using the transversal technique. For approximately 30 seconds, the tip of the brush containing the gel should be rubbed over the tooth surfaces of a hemiarch, exerting light pressure on the proximal and occlusal surfaces. Start with the upper right hemiarch and, in a clockwise direction, repeat the procedure to reach the four hemiarchs, totaling 2 minutes of exposure to the gel. Instruct the child not to swallow it under any circumstances (Cury *et al.*, 2007).

The purpose of this activity is only to apply fluoride, therefore it is not to brush the teeth. Therefore, the person applying the fluoride is not the child, but the agent of the action. It is recommended that no more than 6 children be called at the same time to apply the fluoride gel, in order to facilitate the flow. It is extremely important that this number is not exceeded, since the fluoride content present in gels is very high, and it is necessary to have absolute control over the use of the product in children, so that the teeth will not be brushed, but rather the fluoride will be applied with the bristles of the toothbrush. It is strongly recommended that children, or even unqualified adults, should not be allowed to handle fluorinated gel (Cury *et al.*, 2007).

Fluoride Varnish Application Technique: Although the amount of fluoride reagent in fluoride varnishes is approximately 23,000 ppm F, its adhesiveness allows it to be applied only to the areas of greatest risk, minimizing exposure to a high amount of fluoride. For this reason, it is the most indicated fluoride vehicle for babies at high risk of caries (and for other individuals as well). This varnish is applied in a clinical environment, with the aid of brushes, and there are no descriptions of application techniques in collective environments (Cury *et al.*, 2007).

However, the indication that, at 18 years of age, adolescents consider themselves to be unfit to maintain their own oral health, due to economic limitations and weaknesses in oral health education activities, was considered unsatisfactory and doubtful (Cangassu & Costa, 2001).

4.1.3 Fluoridated water

The worldwide addition of fluoride to public water supplies began in the first half of the 20th century, when the American dentist Frederick McKay demonstrated the activity of the fluoride ion, in the ideal and safe concentration, in preventing tooth decay.

Fluoridation of public water supplies (FAAP) is one of the most comprehensive measures for preventing and controlling dental caries, as it has a large population reach and is the safest, most effective, simple and economical method for preventing dental caries, reducing the prevalence of this disease in people of different social levels. The adoption of this measure has been a recommendation insistently reiterated by international and national organizations in the health sector (Basting *et al.*, 1997; Ramires & Buzalaf, 2007).

In Brazil, water supply fluoridation began in 1953 in the city of Baixo Guandu in Espírito Santo. This supply system was operated by the SESP Foundation of the Ministry of Health, through the regular concentration of fluoride ions in the public water supply, and achieved a reduction of around 60% in the activity of tooth decay. After this, a large number of studies developed in different countries corroborate that the ideal dosage of fluoride in drinking water is between 0.7 and 1.2 mg /liter or parts per million of fluoride, always being added in a controlled manner, aiming to achieve concentrations that provide its effective action against tooth decay (Cardoso *et al.*, 2003; Bleicher & Frota, 2006; Lodi *et al.*, 2006).

The pioneering country in water fluoridation was the United States in 1945, followed shortly after by Sweden and West Germany in 1952. In Brazil, water fluoridation has been provided for by federal law since 1974, by federal law number 6050, which establishes the obligation of fluoridation and determines that projects aimed at the construction or expansion of supply systems, where there is a treatment plant, must include provisions and plans on water fluoridation. There is support from national financing programs and the support of generations of health professionals involved in its defense. However, it still only reaches a little more than half of the population (Bleicher & Frota, 2006; Lodi *et al.*, 2006).

Fluoridated water in public water supplies has two positive aspects: treated water and the epidemiological impact on reducing the prevalence and severity of dental caries. Studies show that, in isolation, exposure to other sources of fluoride (such as toothpaste) and access to fluoridated public water supplies guarantee, on average, a 50 a60% reduction in the severity of dental caries lesions, measured by the DMFT index. This shows that the benefits achieved far outweigh the risks of fluorosis, its main side effect. However, the combination of different forms of fluoride use has been identified as one of the main causes of fluorosis incidence (Silva & Maltz, 2001; Menezes *et al.*, 2002).

Fluoridation of public drinking water was seen as the closest public health measure to the ideal for controlling dental caries, since the benefits can transcend all races, ethnicities, and socioeconomic and religious differences. For this reason, water fluoridation is considered one of the most important factors responsible for the decline in dental caries during the second half of the 20th century, and also presents the best cost-benefit ratio of all preventive methods. In Brazil, adding fluoride to tap water costs approximately R$ 1.00 (one Real) per inhabitant per year (Programa Brasil Sorridente. Informativo 2004; Feb./Mar.), an aspect that contributes to the considerable reduction in the costs of dental services after the implementation of this measure. However, in order to reduce dental caries, fluoridation must be continuous and uninterrupted. The maintenance of fluoride levels is necessary due to the action of this ion in the demineralization and remineralization processes that constantly occur in the oral cavity, since the effect of the anticariogenic activity of fluoridated water results mainly from the topical action of fluoride (Rina, 1993; Garcia, 1989; Marthaler, 2003).

External control is the health surveillance of fluoride concentrations carried out by any public or private agency or institution other than the company responsible for the treatment and addition of fluoride to water. In this sense, external control has been motivated to ensure the effectiveness of water fluoridation in controlling dental caries, as well as to prevent episodes of dental fluorosis (Schneider *et al.*, 1992; Pelletier, 2004).

In Brazil, one of the reasons that fully justifies the adoption of water fluoridation is that, in addition to being economically justifiable, the measure benefits those who need it most, since its preventive impact is greater precisely in the population groups with the worst socioeconomic conditions. Therefore, not fluoridating water in Brazil or interrupting its continuity should be considered a legally illegal attitude (Law No. 6,050/74), scientifically unsustainable and socially unjust (Brazil, 2015).

In 2004, the federal government reported that 40 million Brazilians benefited from water fluoridation (Programa Brasil Sorridente. Informativo 2004; Feb./Mar.) and Brazil's oral health guidelines indicated that water fluoridation was a government priority, through the Programa Brasil Sorridente – water fluoridation subcomponent (Brazil, 2015).

Access to fluoridated public water supplies should be universal. However, there are situations in which this does not happen, whether in rural communities or even in some urban areas. Water fluoridation has been carried out as a complement to the treatment process of water intended for public supply in several municipalities in the country. This is used with the aim of reducing dental caries in the population and is practiced in 45.7% of Brazilian municipalities. The highest rates of application of the procedure are in the Southeast and South regions, where 70% of the respective municipalities systematically distribute fluoridated water. However, only 7.82% of all municipalities in the North region add fluoride to the water, highlighting the great disparity that exists in the national territory (Graph 1) (IBGE, 2000).

State/Region	Total municipalities	Total number of municipalities with water distribution network	Total number of municipalities that add fluoride to distributed water	% of municipalities that add fluoride to distributed water
NORTH	449	422	33	7.82
NORTH EAST	1,787	1,722	285	16.55
SOUTHEAST	1,666	1,666	1,167	70.05
SOUTH	1,159	1,142	799	69.96
C. WEST	446	439	182	41.46
BRAZIL	5,507	5.391	2,466	45.74

Table 1. Total number of Brazilian municipalities, Brazilian municipalities with a water distribution network, Brazilian municipalities that add fluoride to the distribution network by geographic region

Source: IBGE, 2000

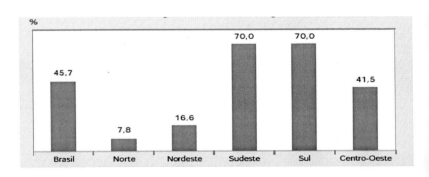

Graph 1. Proportion of municipalities supplied with fluoridated water, according to the Major Regions

Source: IBGE, 2000

4.1.4 Fluoridated toothpaste

The fluoride in fluoridated toothpastes maintains the mineral balance of the teeth, interfering with the initiation and progression of caries lesions. In addition, it activates the remineralizing capacity of saliva, controlled by the cleaning effect (brushing, removal of bacterial plaque, action of saliva) and the action of fluoride (remineralizing and preventive effect) (Rouxel *et al.*, 2008).

Fluoridated toothpaste is an effective means of preventing tooth decay and is also the most widely used method for topical self-application of fluorides, and can be applied in preventive programs in communities and schools. Due to the multifactorial etiology of tooth decay, brushing with toothpaste causes the release of fluorides and also the disorganization of the biofilm, thus this method has come to be considered the method of choice for the prevention of this disease. There are several factors that determine the effectiveness of toothpaste, such as: fluoride concentration, amount of paste on the brush, brushing frequency, time of brushing, among others (Rouxel *et al.*, 2008; Tenuta *et al.*, 2010).

The market offers conventional toothpastes with 1000 to 1100 ppm of fluoride in their composition and high-concentration ones with 1450 a1500 ppm, which have specific indications. And a fluoridated toothpaste for babies was recently launched in Brazil that contains a reduced concentration of fluoride (500 ppm) (Chedid, 1999).

However, regardless of the need, tartar control, whitening, fresh breath, among others, experts are unanimous in saying that fluoride is one of the fundamental principles of the product. According to the Academy of General Dentistry (ADA), in the United States, brushing your teeth with fluoride toothpaste twice a day is enough to reduce the appearance of cavities by 40%.

Daily use is one of the main factors responsible for reducing tooth decay rates, due to the topical action of fluoride in the oral cavity. According to SNVS Ordinance No. 71 of May 29, 1996 – some of which had its annexes revoked by Resolution No. 79 of August 28, 2000 –, commercial toothpastes are not required to contain fluoride, but if they do, they must comply with the recommendations regarding the type and characteristics of the fluoride compound. Toothpastes are also used in collective actions as a vehicle for topical fluoride during supervised toothbrushing. This activity must be performed at least quarterly for all individuals, regardless of the risk group they are part of (Chedid, 1999).

It is very important to know the correct amount of toothpaste to use for each brushing. For babies under 3 years of age, it is recommended to use toothpastes without fluoride, which can be purchased at pharmacies, or to use toothpastes with fluoride in very small and careful quantities. If you choose to use toothpaste with fluoride, you should fill a modified baby toothbrush one third full, using the cap technique, the amount deposited on the cap after pressing the closed tube or the equivalent of a grain of canary seed (Chedid, 1999).

The amount of toothpaste for preschool children should be equivalent to a pea, using the transversal technique, or 0,5 gby brushing. After 8 years of age, the longitudinal technique can be used, 1 gby brushing (Villena, Ando, 1995).

Toothpastes with less than 600 ppm are recommended for children under 7 years of age, who have a low risk of cavities, living in municipalities with fluoridated water (Rouxel *et al.*, 2008).

In children at high risk of cavitation, brushing must be supervised by adults. Concentrations of 1000 ppm to 1500 ppm can be used in individuals over 6 years of age (Rouxel *et al.*, 2008).

Children aged 2 to 4 years swallow, on average, 50% of the toothpaste used for brushing their teeth. For children aged 5 to 7 years, this percentage is less than 25%. This is a proven risk factor for dental fluorosis. To prevent the problem, parents or guardians should be instructed to supervise brushing at home or in group settings, at least until the child is 7 years old, to instruct the child not to swallow the toothpaste used for brushing, and to apply a small amount of toothpaste to the brush. The recommended technique for use is the transverse technique (Albuquerque *et al.*, 2003).

ABO, as well as the Ministry of Health, recommends the use of conventional toothpaste with fluoride from the eruption of the first deciduous molars (around 14 months), in a quantity equivalent to a grain of raw rice, and should be carried out by parents or caregivers, between one and three times a day, depending on the parents' availability.

There are some toothpastes on the market that, instead of fluoride, use products such as chlorhexidine, xylitol and mallow. Toothpaste with xylitol has the ability to treat and prevent cavities, but it is more expensive and requires more research. Mallow has anti-inflammatory and antimicrobial action, but it also needs more studies. Chlorhexidine is indicated for specific cases of risk of cavities, but this product can cause the appearance of external stains on the teeth. The recommendation of the Brazilian Association of Pediatric Dentistry is that parents seek guidance from a pediatric dentist so that the professional can assess the child's individual needs and determine the curative or preventive treatment.

Before the baby's teeth appear, use only a clean cloth or gauze moistened with filtered water or saline solution. You should clean your baby's gums thoroughly. After the first tooth appears, you can brush your baby's teeth, but do not use toothpaste, unless your baby's dentist recommends it for some reason.

When brushing, put the equivalent of a grain of rice (0.1g) of toothpaste on the toothbrush of babies and children who cannot spit, and the equivalent of a pea (0.3g) for children who can spit. Brushing with this amount of fluoride toothpaste should be done two or three times a day, to avoid exceeding the recommended safe dose. The ideal toothpaste for children should contain 1,000 to 1,100 ppm of sodium fluoride (fluoride) to protect against cavities.

Transverse Technique: consists of placing the toothpaste tube in a perpendicular position along the axis of the brush and dispensing in the center of the active tip of the instrument a quantity of toothpaste corresponding to, at most, half the width of the active tip. This quantity is generally equivalent to a grain of small pea and is sufficient for the purpose. This technique is also recommended for adolescents and adults (Vilhena *et al.,* 2008).

To further reduce the amount of toothpaste to be used on children under 4 years of age (since they ingest larger quantities), the cap technique is suggested.

Cap Technique: Take the closed tube and press the tube lightly so that a small amount of toothpaste is retained on the inside of the cap (whether it is screw-on or not). Then, open the tube and press the active tip of the toothbrush against the inside of the cap to transfer the small amount of toothpaste retained there to the toothbrush. This amount is sufficient to deliver the necessary fluoride and to produce the other effects of the toothpaste. This technique is recommended for the first years of life and up to approximately 4 years of age (Vilhena *et al.,* 2008).

When recommending the use of fluoride for preschoolers, it is essential to first analyze the risk of tooth decay for that patient, so that prevention can be achieved appropriately and the possibility of fluorosis or fluoride poisoning can be ruled out (Chankanka *et al.,* 2010).

Other toothpastes contain triclosan as an active ingredient. This substance works by combating gum inflammation, which is why it is recommended for people with gingivitis.

Some toothpastes contain substances that combat tooth sensitivity. There are several compounds that act with this function. Some even have immediate effects. In short, they act by obliterating the dental canals, preventing sensitivity from occurring.

Some toothpastes combine several compounds, so ask your dentist which is best for you.

The famous toothpastes that claim to be whitening, bleaching (or whitening) are actually nothing more than toothpastes with a higher abrasive content, which promote a greater polishing of the tooth surface. They do not change its color per se. Therefore, they do not have the potential to whiten the teeth intrinsically. For this, the recommended treatment is teeth whitening done under the supervision of a dentist. Whitening toothpastes – like all other toothpastes – contain mild abrasives that help remove stains from the surface of the teeth. However, the shape of the particles used in whitening toothpastes is modified so that they clean better, so there is a noticeable difference in the appearance of your teeth. The toothpastes do not contain bleaches, which makes it impossible to whiten your teeth drastically.

4.1.5 Fluoride supplementation (tablets, tablets or medications)

The use of systemic fluoride supplementation was a method developed for the prevention of dental caries, replacing the fluoridation of public water supplies (Pendrys, 1995). However, it is often used inappropriately, concomitantly with other systemic methods or in excess dosage, constituting a potential risk factor for dental fluorosis in the first eight years of life (Nowjack-Raymer, 1995; Pendrys, 1995; Wang, 1997).

Ismail and Bandekar (1999) identified, in a meta-analysis, that most cross-sectional and case-control studies demonstrate a 1.3 to 10.7 times greater risk of developing dental fluorosis when submitted to supplementation, in areas with non-fluoridated water. In longitudinal studies, this risk was 5 to 15 times greater in this same association.

Therefore, there is a need for additional care when indicating this method: only in high-risk children – low socioeconomic and educational level that hinders access to other topical methods; high level of sugar intake and children of mothers with high activity/risk of caries – and in isolated populations. In addition, it is necessary to provide broad information to other health professionals about the availability of other systemic fluoride methods offered to the community (Horowitz, 1996; Ismail & Bandekar, 1999; Levy, 1995; Nowjack-Raymer, 1995; Wang, 1997).

4.1.6 Fluoride ingested in the diet

There are several foods and beverages available in the diet that contain high levels of fluoride and are associated with the presence of dental fluorosis – fish, shellfish, chicken (when fed with bone meal), teas, as well as beverages, infant formulas and milk when processed in regions with fluoridated public water supply (Clarck *et al.*, 1994; Gonini, 1999; Horowitz, 1996; Levy, 1995).

It is also observed that children are increasingly consuming processed foods, soft drinks and powdered milk, accompanied by a reduction in the consumption of water and milk from other sources, which significantly increases the systemic intake of fluoride at an age when there is a greater risk of fluorosis. However, it is still difficult to measure the amount of fluoride intake through diet, due to methodological difficulties in measuring individual levels of fluoride in each food in the active form, the amount ingested and the total amount absorbed by the tissues (Brothwell & Limeback, 1999; Heller, 1999).

Villena *et al.* (1996), in a study conducted with 104 commercial brands of mineral water manufactured in Brazil, reported that 7.7% of them contained levels above 1 ppm of fluoride. In this sense, it is necessary to reinforce health surveillance actions, such as reducing the fluoride content in manufactured baby foods; to regulate the mandatory labeling of fluoride concentrations, and for these to be done in a standardized manner (Levy, 1995; Villena *et al.*, 1996); and to implement health education actions that enable the population to assimilate and interpret the available information (Horowitz, 1995).

4.2 Creation of a global oral health campaign. Black March

World Oral Health Day, celebrated on March 20, was created to raise awareness about the importance of oral hygiene and preventing dental problems. It is worth remembering once again that it is the third most prevalent disease and that it worsens and develops a series of other diseases. It is really important to reevaluate and give due importance to this issue, which can save thousands of people. Because a person without teeth does not eat properly, as they are unable to chew more solid foods, such as protein, and will suffer from malnutrition, aggravating other systemic diseases. A diabetic or hypertensive person may only eat soft foods and foods with sugar, such as fast-absorbing carbohydrates, causing hyperglycemic spikes that will be harmful to their body.

In this way, we support the application of topical fluoride and sealant to children and adolescents on this day. We provide toothbrushing kits and teach toothbrushing techniques to mitigate dental problems in everyday life and in the future, which can be aggravated nutritionally, causing problems such as worsening of general clinical conditions of chronic diseases.

However, just one day is not enough. It would be better to create a strong and active campaign throughout the month of March, which would bring the media and people around the world to the attention and prevention of this widespread and common disease.

Tooth decay is often considered one of the most prevalent diseases in the world. According to the World Health Organization (WHO) and other public health sources, tooth decay affects a large proportion of the global population, regardless of age. It is a common dental condition and can affect people of all ages, from infants to the elderly.

The prevalence of dental caries is high mainly due to factors such as a diet high in sugars, lack of adequate oral hygiene and limited access to dental care in some regions. Despite advances in prevention and treatment, dental caries remains a significant public health problem globally.

Dental caries is extremely common but is often not listed as a leading cause of mortality or morbidity in global reports because it is not often fatal and can be managed with treatment and preventative care. However, it often masquerades as other diseases and greatly aggravates them.

Therefore, it is certainly among the most common conditions affecting health globally, especially when considering its high incidence and the impact it has on people's quality of life and oral health.

Carry out a month-long campaign worldwide, such as Black March, which automatically brings to mind a pathology that is very common, highly prevalent and has strong painful symptoms, being one of the worst types of pain that can be witnessed, second only to heart attacks, renal colic, childbirth and burns (Hortense & Souza, 2009). Associated with other campaigns that use a month with a strong color, such as black. As an example, we have Pink October, a month to raise awareness about breast cancer, which is of unparalleled importance, but the rates of caries (the third most prevalent disease in the world) are immense and also cause associated or unrelated mortality, often undiagnosed by health professionals and lay people themselves, due to lack of knowledge and the lack of dentists in multidisciplinary teams in hospitals around the world. This is a well-established practice in several centers, and we also created and developed it at the Check Up Hospital in Manaus, a pioneering initiative in northern Brazil.

Using high-resolution computed tomography with specific visualization by software and a medical radiology team trained to provide details about the bone and dental quality of this patient, combining blood tests with clinical dental practice, elucidating cases that were previously not closed in their diagnosis.

The month of March was chosen because World Oral Health Day is March 20th, and black, a strong and shocking color, can draw attention to an unnecessarily neglected subject, reminding us of the color of tooth decay, which causes pain, infection and necrosis of dental tissue. These measures would bring more attention to oral health for health professionals and also for the entire world population. It would be a great ally in the fight against tooth decay and oral diseases.

5

DISCUSSION

Narvai (1998) discusses health surveillance and oral health in Brazil. He begins the article by discussing the different concepts of health surveillance, but makes it clear that the formulators of these concepts always agree on the fundamental role of the State in this area. The author continues by directing the subject to oral health and states that health surveillance actions are changing focus, since there is a shift in actions from the dental office to the environment, considered in a broad sense. He states that in the context of collective oral health and the area of dental practice, health surveillance actions cover three dimensions: establishments providing dental services, food and beverages, and oral hygiene products. In relation to these, the following are mentioned: toothbrushes, dental floss, and fluoridated toothpastes. The latter are considered the main fluoridated products, since they are used by practically the entire world population. According to the author, more than 5 billion tubes of toothpaste are consumed annually throughout the world. Fluoride present in toothpaste is considered the main agent of interest in terms of health surveillance, and it has been proven that the presence of this ion is associated with a lower incidence of dental caries in the population. The author makes clear the importance of toothpaste containing reactive fluoride and also the need for products to present information regarding the chemical formula of the fluoride compound used, its concentration in ppm, the respective indications, how to use it, the date of manufacture and the expiration date. For this reason, it is important to control and monitor these products, with the aim of being effective in terms of promoting the health of the population.

Narvai (2000), through a review, analyzed the binomial dental caries and fluoride: a relationship from the 20th century. Initially, the author presents a historical context and gives the names of researchers who have entered the history of public health. Then, he talks about dental caries and the human eating pattern over the years. Later, the author instructs about fluoride, fluoridated water and water fluoridation.

The author highlights the importance of the mechanism of action of topical fluoride and fluoridated toothpaste. With regard to this fluoride vehicle, until the 1960s it had a merely cosmetic role, and was later elevated to the category of preventive agent. The author explains that at the end of the century, practically all toothpastes sold in Brazil contained fluoride ion and that the consumption of this product has been increasing in recent years.

It also reveals the importance of quality control of fluoridated products sold in the country, since the population needs active fluoride to intervene in the process of tooth decay. Therefore, health surveillance of fluoride is important, both in relation to fluoridated toothpastes and in relation to water fluoridation. Finally, the author summarizes that the use of fluoride, especially through fluoridated toothpastes, has made it possible to benefit millions of people, freeing them from tooth decay or reducing the severity of this disease.

5.1 Controversy

There are some questions about the fluoride used in water leading to the emergence of several organic and mental problems in human beings.

Fluoride is widely regarded as a life-sustaining trace element, functioning primarily as a protection against dental caries, and also playing a role in bone mineralization. However, excess fluoride can be harmful to the human body. Recently, researchers have noted that fluoride toxicity appears to begin in the fetal stage (Daijei, 1984; Zhongzhong, 1987).

He *et al.* (2008) report specimens of induced abortions in fluoride-endemic and unaffected areas, and, through histochemical analysis, enzymatic-chemical analysis, light microscopy and electron microscopy, investigate the effects of fluoride on the fetus, providing evidence that in early childhood there is a possibility of fluorosis. These findings indicate that neurons in the cerebral cortex of the developing brain may be one of the targets of fluoride.

While 49 studies found an association between fluoride and IQ, the following seven studies found no such association. There are several points to consider about these studies.

First, a new study from New Zealand (Broadbent, 2014) reports no association between fluoridation and IQ. As acknowledged by Dr. Philippe Grandjean in 2019, however, there are several glaring problems with this study, including the fact that virtually all of the children in the "non-fluoridated" community had not used fluoride supplements (a prescription medication designed to provide the same amount of fluoride that a child would get from drinking fluoridated water). Fan discusses these problems here.

Second, Calderon's (2000) study found that fluoride exposure was associated with other indices of neurotoxicity, including impaired visuospatial organization.

Third, Li's (2010) study did not compare a high fluoride area against a low fluoride area. Instead, he compared the IQ of children with dental fluorosis in a high fluoride area with the IQ of children without dental fluorosis in the same high fluoride area.

Fourth, Spittle's (1998) study of a fluoridated community in New Zealand made no attempt to determine children's urinary fluoride levels. This is particularly important to do in studies of Western populations, because there is now a great deal of overlap in fluoride exposures between children living in non-fluoridated *vs.* fluoridated communities. This overlap in exposure is due to several factors, including: (1) frequent prescription of fluoride supplements to children in non-fluoridated areas; (2) ingestion of large quantities of fluoridated toothpaste; (3) exposure to fluoridated water through processed foods and beverages; (4) exposure to fluoride through pesticides; and (5) exposure to fluoride from Teflon. Thus, any study of IQ in Western populations that does not include a measure of the individual's fluoride exposure will be unlikely to find an association between fluoride and IQ.

For years, health experts have been unable to agree on whether fluoride in drinking water can be toxic to the developing human brain. Extremely high levels of fluoride are known to cause neurotoxicity in adults, and negative impacts on memory and learning have been reported in rodent studies, but little is known about the substance's impact on neurodevelopment in children. In a meta-analysis, researchers from the Harvard School of Public Health (HSPH) and China Medical University in Shenyang for the first time combined 27 studies and found strong evidence that fluoride can negatively affect cognitive development in children. Based on the results, the authors say this risk should not be ignored, and that more research on fluoride's impact on the developing brain is needed.

The study was published online in *Environmental Health Perspectives* on July 20, 2012.

The researchers conducted a systematic review of studies, nearly all of which came from China, where the risks of fluoride are well established. Fluoride is a naturally occurring substance in groundwater, and concerns about the chemical are heightened in some parts of China. There are virtually no human studies in this field, with only those conducted in the U.S., said lead author Anna Choi, a research scientist in the Department of Environmental Health at HSPH.

Even though many of the studies on children in China differed in many ways or were incomplete, the authors consider the data collection and pooled analysis an important first step in assessing potential risk. "For the first time, we have been able to do a comprehensive meta-analysis that has the potential to help us design better studies. We want to make sure that cognitive development is considered as a possible target for fluoride toxicity," said Choi *et al.* (2012).

Choi and senior author Philippe Grandjean, an associate professor of environmental health at HSPH, and their colleagues reviewed epidemiological studies of children exposed to fluoride in drinking water in 2019. The China National Knowledge Infrastructure database was also used to locate studies published in Chinese journals. They then analyzed possible associations with IQ measures in more than 8,000 school-aged children; one study suggested that high fluoride levels in water may negatively affect cognitive development.

The average IQ loss was reported as a standardized weighted mean difference of 0.45, which would be approximately equivalent to seven IQ points for commonly used IQ scores with a standard deviation of 15. Some studies have suggested that even a slight increase in fluoride exposure may be toxic to the brain. Thus, children in areas of high fluoride concentration had significantly lower IQ scores than those living in areas of low fluoride concentration. The children studied were up to 14 years of age, but the researchers speculate that any toxic effects on brain development may have occurred earlier, and that the brain may not be fully able to compensate for the toxicity.

Fluoride seems to fit in with lead, mercury, and other poisons that cause chemical leakage. The effect of each toxic substance may seem small, but the combined damage on a population scale can be severe, especially since the brain power of the next generation is crucial to all of us (Granjean, 2019).

The use of fluoride has promoted significant improvements in oral health and quality of life of populations, through the reduction of dental caries rates (Burt, 1995). However, numerous studies have been published identifying the first clinical sign of the toxic effect of this substance – dental fluorosis (Brothwell & Limeback, 1999; Burt, 1995; Fejerskov, 1994).

There is therefore a need to critically evaluate the existing epidemiological data on dental fluorosis, from the perspective of whether or not it constitutes a relevant public health problem. In addition, the effectiveness and safety of the use of fluoride in its various forms will be discussed, proposing health surveillance actions in order to ensure its maximum benefit without undesirable side effects.

Clinical and epidemiological aspects The causes of dental fluorosis are related to the exposure of the tooth germ, during its formation process, to high concentrations of fluoride ions. As a consequence, there are defects in enamel mineralization, with severity directly associated with the amount ingested. Generally, the clinical aspect is from opaque spots on the enamel, in homologous teeth, to yellowish or brown regions in cases of more severe changes (DenBesten, 1999; Fejerskov, 1994).

In addition to fluoride dosage, other factors affect the severity of the disease: low body weight, skeletal growth rate and bone remodeling periods are phases of greater fluoride absorption; nutritional status, altitude and changes in renal activity and calcium homeostasis are also relevant factors (DenBesten, 1999). In this sense, the disease is more frequent in teeth with late mineralization (permanent dentition), in children with low weight or poor nutritional status or chronic renal failure, with the age groups of early and middle childhood being considered those at greatest risk of systemic fluoride ingestion and, consequently, its harmful effects (Fejerskov, 1994).

Epidemiological studies carried out around the world in the 1990s describe differences in the prevalence of fluorosis, which vary from the near absence of the disease in populations, 2.2%, to proportions greater than 90% (Akpata et al., 1997; Downer, 1994). In general, high prevalences are present where there are natural sources with high fluoride content or ingestion of multiple sources of this ion and, historically, fluorosis has been endemic in all age groups, such as China (Burt, 1995), locations in Africa (El Nadef & Honkala, 1998; Kloss & Haimanot, 1999; N'ang'a & Valderhaug, 1993), Saudi Arabia (Akpata et al., 1997), Singapore (Lo & Bagramian, 1996), United States, Canada, Brazil and Colombia (Azcurra et al., 1995; Clarck et al., 1994; Cortes et al., 1996; Selwitz et al., 1995; Skotowski et al., 1996).

The disease has shown higher prevalence and severity at younger ages in studies in the same location, which has alerted the scientific community to the need for continuous and effective monitoring to detect a possible secular trend of increasing dental fluorosis (Heintze et al., 1998; Levy et al., 1995). However, there is still disagreement between the findings: Selwitz et al. (1995) describe that in Switzerland no evidence of an increase in the prevalence or severity of dental fluorosis was found, while Lewis and Banting (1994) identify in the United States a clear increase of approximately 33% in the prevalence of the disease in regions with fluoridated water and 9% without fluoridated water.

On August 19, 2019, an article published by Rivka Green *et al.* in *JAMA Pediatrics* reported on an epidemiological study conducted in Canada that examined the relationship between pregnant women's exposure to water fluoridation during pregnancy and their children's intelligence quotient (IQ). A decrease in IQ scores was observed with increasing fluoride exposure.

This study was noteworthy because participants lived in communities where water fluoride concentrations were at the level recommended by the United States Public Health Service (0.7 mg of fluoride per liter of water).

The records of 601 mother-child pairs (fluoride intake of pregnant women and IQ scores of their children when they were 3–4 years old) were available for study. Fluoride intake during pregnancy was estimated based on urinary fluoride concentration (measured 3 times during pregnancy in 512 women). Analysis of the data revealed that for every 1 mg increase in urinary fluoride concentration, there was a decrease in IQ points in male children. A similar decrease was not observed in female children. Furthermore, fluoride intake by mothers (based on data from a questionnaire completed twice during pregnancy by 400 women) would reflect the exposure of fathers and children, who presumably drink from the same water source as their mothers. Here, for every 1 mg increase in fluoride, the child's IQ decreased by 3.7 points, and this was observed in both male and female children.

The authors noted that the uniqueness of the findings is the reduced IQ of children living in an area where water was fluoridated to the currently established optimal level. The overall finding of neurotoxic effects of fluoride in water is consistent with other recent studies that have reported reduced neurological function in children exposed to water fluoridation, including reduced memory and learning, IQ 3.4, cognitive development, and a higher prevalence of attention deficit/hyperactivity disorder. A meta-analysis of the association between water fluoridation and children's intelligence concluded that "greater exposure to high levels of fluoride in water was significantly associated with reduced levels of intelligence in children." Other adverse systemic effects of exposure to fluoride in drinking water have been examined, but these associations have not been well defined (Rivka Green *et al.*, 2019).

This recently published paper was expected to be controversial, and two commentaries were published in the same issue of *JAMA Pediatrics* to accompany the research report. The first was a brief editor's note stating that the journal decided to publish the paper even though it acknowledged that the conclusions would be controversial. However, the editor supported the soundness of the research, and the manuscript was reviewed very carefully before publication. Furthermore, the journal's mission is to improve children's health, so it needs to present solid evidence. It also acknowledged that no single study will determine the final answer.

A thoughtful and balanced editorial by Silva *et al.* (2021) also accompanied the published article. In this editorial, several important points were highlighted.

1. Water fluoridation to prevent tooth decay is considered one of the top 10 public health measures of the 20th century.

2. There has always been a minority that has opposed the fluoridation of public water supplies because it represents a mandatory medication administered indiscriminately to water consumers without their consent. Other objections include an increase in the occurrence of dental and skeletal fluorosis (Silva *et al.,* 2021).

3. The quality of previous publications examining the relationship between fluoride exposure and cognition has generally been poor, and not all studies report an inverse relationship.

4. The authors of the *JAMA Pediatrics publication* acknowledged that their research findings would be scrutinized, but their research methodology and statistical analysis were thorough and their conclusions robust.

5. Considering these conclusions, fluoride as a toxicant for neurological development should now be seriously considered (Silva *et al.,* 2021).

6. The need for further research is critical. Many questions remain, including the generalizability of the new findings, what other aspects of cognitive function are affected, and what is the critical period of fetal exposure. It is important to emphasize that this research and subsequent discussion of the results should focus on the reliability of the data.

JAMA Pediatrics article, the American Dental Association issued a press release stating that water fluoridation is the most effective public health approach to preventing tooth decay. It went on to echo themes raised in the editorial. These include the importance of examining all available data, the existing evidence supporting the safety of water fluoridation, and the need to continually evaluate new research findings.

The report by Rivka Green *et al.* (2019) will certainly reignite the debate on the benefits/risks of water fluoridation, a debate that is often rancorous and controversial. It is important to note that other means of delivering fluoride, specifically in different topical forms, have been shown to be very successful in preventing dental caries, namely in toothpastes, mouthwashes and as varnish. Under appropriate conditions, these approaches to topical fluoride delivery are associated with a very small risk of systemic fluoride ingestion.

Oral health care providers need to be aware of the most recent information on this topic. When asked about this research, providers should be familiar with the points made in the original article, as well as the accompanying editorial and the ADA statement. These points include the long history of successful use of water fluoridation to prevent tooth decay, and that a 1 mg change in fluoride concentration in drinking water (the relative change referenced above) represents a very large difference when considering the ideal fluoride concentration in drinking water. The controversy over this issue certainly continues. However, it will never erase what science has determined to be a fact: yes, fluoride is excellent in preventing tooth decay, without having a major effect on other pathologies, as is often associated without scientific basis.

Therefore, in our experience and practice in the state of Amazonas, where we do not have water fluoridation, and observing that the water used in the city of Manaus in Amazonas and throughout the Amazon has a high acidity that causes more cavities throughout the region, coupled with the large amount of simple carbohydrates ingested, causing cavities and infections in the oral cavity, we have still seen an exacerbated increase in cases of autism at all levels and other neurological syndromes. Despite the fact that we have never had any type of fluoridation and there is very little per capita access to fluoride in toothpaste or other possibilities, we can know that there really are other aspects to be considered and not just blaming fluoride, which saves so many mouths from cavities or tooth extractions.

The unregulated and unsupervised mining of precious minerals, including gold, with the use of mercury and other heavy metals, widespread in the Amazon, extremely profitable, with contamination of fish and organisms, this can indeed cause gigantic effects on the health of human beings, even neurologically. But corrupt and unprepared governments prefer to place the blame on other situations, which make no sense. Manipulating the people in a vicious and eternal cycle of lack of health and education, remaining longer and longer in government, stealing and destroying society.

5.2 Fluoride and its mode of action

Fluoride has been shown to be a therapeutic agent that modulates dental caries. Frequent contact between patients and small concentrations of fluoride hinders demineralization and activates remineralization, in addition to inhibiting cariogenic microorganisms. Controlling the patient's caries activity is the initial phase of restorative treatment. To achieve this, basic procedures for conditioning or adapting the oral environment are necessary to reduce infection levels and mineral losses. Mass excavation of cavitated carious lesions with removal of all carious tissue from the dentinal-enamel junction, infected and disorganized dentin, and temporary sealing of these cavities with iono-meric cements not only contribute to the process of adaptation to the proposed objectives, but also enable the remineralization of the adjacent dental tissue underlying the provisional restoration, and block the metabolic circuit of the remaining bacteria with the oral environment, paralyzing the carious lesion (Cury, 1992; Liporoni, 1995; Maia & Valença, 1995; Ten Cate & Van Duinen, 1995; Harari, 1996; Modesto & Primo, 1996; Kramer, 1997; Noronha, 2024).

Topical fluoride applications in the dental office are part of oral conditioning and can be performed weekly, biweekly or monthly, depending on the patient's needs in terms of mineral loss observed by the amount of active white spots present. Therefore, the applied fluoride will interfere with the enamel demineralization process, inactivating and reversing it, with weekly applications of acidulated fluorophosphate at 1.23%. However, it is necessary to observe whether the patient has composite restorations, in which case the option will be neutral gel fluoride, due to the compromise of the surface resistance of these restorations by the action of acidulated fluoride (Liporoni, 1995; Maia & Valença, 1995; Andrade et al., 1996).

In topical fluoride fluoridation, there is evidence that the effectiveness of acidulated phosphate fluoride ranges from 20-30% to 30-50% in reducing the prevalence of caries. However, its indiscriminate use, especially by young people, can lead to toxicity. Therefore, research was conducted to evaluate the safest and most effective method of topical application (Barros et al., 2008).

After more than 50 years of fluoridation of public water supplies in Brazil, many studies have been conducted to evaluate the benefits of fluoridation through epidemiological studies on the prevalence of caries, as well as the harmful effects of fluoridation, mainly represented by dental fluorosis. The CEO-d and DMFT indices found in epidemiological surveys of 1986, 1996 and 2003, carried out by the Ministry of Health, as well as a study carried out by SESI in 1993, showed that the prevalence of caries has been decreasing, suggesting that the incorporation of fluoride in water, together with other oral health prevention programs, as well as the use of fluoridated toothpastes, played an important role in this result (Basting *et al.*, 1997; Gomes *et al.*, 2004; Hoffmann *et al.*, 2004).

Sales-Peres *et al.* (2002) did not observe a statistically significant difference between the prevalence of caries in municipalities with or without fluoridated water. In a similar study, but with different results, Cypriano *et al.* (2003) observed a slight decrease in the prevalence of caries in places without fluoridated water and a much lower prevalence in places with fluoridated water.

The WHO targets for the year 2000, which serve as a reference for assessing the severity of caries worldwide, were achieved in almost all of these studies that presented fluoride in their public water supplies. The age group of 12 years was the one that most achieved the DMFT target, which was approximately 3.0 (Basting *et al.*, 1997; Gomes *et al.*, 2004; Hoffmann *et al.*, 2004).

For Campos *et al.* (1998), Cypriano *et al.* (2003) and the Ministry of Health (2003), the prevalence of dental fluorosis has been low and mild in places with public water supply fluoridation. The percentage among most of the authors surveyed ranged from 7.9% to 20%.

Although there is a low prevalence of fluorosis in many places with fluoridated water, continuous external control of the concentration of fluoride incorporated into the water supply is important to support the justification that fluoride in water is in fact an efficient method in the prevention and control of dental caries (Maia *et al.*, 2003; Lima *et al.*, 2004; Silva *et al.*, 2007).

In Brazil, water fluoridation in public supplies has full support, especially from the federal government, since in the 1970s a law was enacted requiring the fluoridation of public water supplies where there are water treatment systems, standardizing the construction and expansion of water treatment plants and operationalizing water fluoridation (Brazil, 1974; Santa Catarina, 1982). In the state of São Paulo, the fluoride concentration is in accordance with the recommendations of the Ministry of Health ordinance (São Paulo, 1995). Therefore, for there to be correct fluoridation of public water supplies, there must be surveillance, control and procedural methods for implementation, and there must be greater control by the federal, state and municipal governments, with due guidance from the Ministry of Health (Lima *et al.,* 2004; Silva *et al.,* 2007).

5.3 Considerations on fluoride, health and oral infections not diagnosed by health professionals, which cause mortality in many patients

After such extensive clinical and academic experience reaching so many patients from all socioeconomic classes, as previously described, awareness about this important issue has become more present in our lives, creating the dream of zero cavities in the world, but this will only be achieved with the support of public policies, family members and health professionals, with knowledge and pro-health action.

Fluoride has been widely studied and is recognized for its role in preventing tooth decay. It strengthens tooth enamel and helps prevent demineralization, which reduces the incidence of cavities. Fluoride is added to many toothpastes and, in some places, to drinking water in safe concentrations to benefit public dental health.

However, there is ongoing debate about the potential adverse effects of fluoride when used in excess. Excessive use can lead to dental fluorosis, a condition that causes stains or streaks on the teeth, but at normal, controlled levels, fluoride is generally considered safe and beneficial.

5.4 Oral Health and Undiagnosed Infections

Undiagnosed or inadequately treated oral infections can have serious consequences for overall health. Some dental infections, such as abscesses, can spread to other parts of the body and cause serious complications, such as endocarditis (infection of the heart valves) or septicemia (generalized blood infection). These conditions can, in fact, be fatal if not treated in time. And when associated with other chronic diseases, they are sometimes confused by doctors due to the lack of study in the global scope of Dentistry in association with Medicine, since the human body is only one and all sciences must come together with the purpose of improving the quality of life for the patient.

5.5 Challenges in Detection and Diagnosis

1. **Delayed Diagnosis:** Mouth infections can sometimes be difficult to detect early, especially in the early stages, and may not present clear symptoms until the condition has worsened.
2. **Lack of Access:** In some areas, access to dental care may be limited, and many patients may not have the follow-up care needed to identify and treat oral problems before they become serious.
3. **Ambiguous Symptoms:** Some infections may have symptoms that are confused with other conditions, making rapid diagnosis difficult.

5.6 Importance of Preventive Care

1. **Proper Oral Hygiene:** Maintaining good oral hygiene is essential. Brushing your teeth regularly, flossing, and visiting your dentist regularly can help prevent serious problems.
2. **Regular Checkups:** Regular dental checkups are important to detect and treat oral problems before they become serious. Imaging tests and clinical evaluations can help identify infections that are not visible to the naked eye.
3. **Education and Awareness:** Education about the importance of oral health and early detection of symptoms are crucial. Patients should be aware of the signs of dental infections and seek appropriate medical treatment when necessary.

In short, fluoride, when used correctly, plays an important role in dental health and preventing cavities. However, oral health involves much more than just applying fluoride. Early detection and treatment of oral infections are essential to preventing serious complications and improving overall health.

In these more than 70 years of clinical and academic experience, we have seen that health professionals in general do not understand the complexity and systemic impact on patients and public health in general. This leads to absolute disregard for dentistry, which is forgotten and sometimes treated in a way that belittles science itself. Perhaps due to a lack of knowledge on the part of many other health professionals. So it is a fact that positions need to change once and for all. Because dentists are seeking their place, I experience this day after day, explaining to other health professionals why dentistry is important and often diagnosing cases of infection without a diagnosis in hospitals. These are in fact diseases in the oral cavity that are killing and causing various physical problems for patients, which cannot be neglected due to the lack of a truly effective multidisciplinary team, with all health professionals working together, as we do at the Check Up Hospital in Manaus, Amazonas, mentioned above.

Working as the head of Dentistry at Hospital Check Up since 2012, which specializes in highly complex cardiological and neurological procedures, we have been working for over 10 years to raise awareness among the multidisciplinary health care team, which has been a fantastic and innovative experience. Transforming patient care into something universal, something that is still very incipient in Brazil and other developed countries around the world. In which we combine cutting-edge diagnostics such as computed tomography with a Medical-Dental focus, blood tests, combining cardiology, neurology, clinical medicine with the services of a dental clinic and oral and maxillofacial surgery. In addition to physiotherapy, speech therapy and psychology. All health sciences promoting the best possible treatment for the patient. However, medical health plans have the view that dental procedures such as tooth extractions and surgical debridement should not be performed by them. Thinking only of the patient without the oral cavity, which would not cause infections or cause death to the patient.

This work also aims to scientifically support the idea that the mouth is obviously part of the human body and that it does indeed require the expansion of the spectrum of health plans on this absolutely important topic, as many patients die today from untreated infections that aggravate thousands of other pathologies, from chronic to acute.

We have already evaluated many cases of bacterial endocarditis caused by the negligence of the patient, who did not seek out the dentist, and of the medical professional, who never looked into the mouth and has no idea of the seriousness of a simple cavity that can develop and cause sepsis, for example, due to the lack of university curricula and syllabuses that can bring together all health sciences to analyze the patient as a whole. For that patient with a chronic disease treated for years did not have a definitive diagnosis of an intraoral infection by the doctor and even due to the patient's own lack of Health Education, which could have been avoided by medical recommendation, which in the vast majority of cases does not indicate dental evaluation in patients.

All this misinformation culminates in cases of reinfection of heart valves or medical stents by bacterial endocarditis, in which the infectious focus is in the mouth and not in other organs in the body, reinfecting an extremely expensive and difficult heart surgery. Everything could be avoided if there were brushing with fluoride and drinking water with an adequate amount of fluoride, application of sealant and adequate brushing. And global oral health campaigns, such as our proposal for Black March, since it is of utmost importance for everyone.

If health plans made correct assessments and without mistaken financial biases, they would understand that dental procedures, before, during or after medical hospitalizations, serious or not, with correct medical assessment evaluating the conduct and possible benefit to the patient, would save millions of dollars or reais, since a cardiac stent costs 10 thousand reais (2 thousand dollars), or a heart valve sometimes costs 50 thousand reais (10 thousand dollars), not including the surgical part, while a tooth extraction procedure would cost one thousand reais, and could prevent other hospitalizations and more complex surgeries, which we know can reach millions of reais or even dollars (all these figures are estimates).

Therefore, highlighting these details is absolutely important, and preventing cavities once again is unquestionable. Once again, it is necessary to bring together doctors, dentists, physiotherapists, pharmacists, nurses, etc., so that the patient is referred and treated correctly.

Billions of reais are often spent on possible biologically active "vaccines" with inactivated *Streptococcus mutans bacteria* or recombinant RNA, which can cause several unknown adverse effects. This will not erase the fact that the mouth is the most infected place in the entire human organism, where we put our hands, objects and food, logically with microorganisms, or kiss our wives, for example, and transmit that microbiota to another person and vice versa.

It is very difficult to eliminate tooth decay itself, as the person will need to brush their teeth for periodontal (gum) reasons and many other reasons. Consequently, it is much easier and more accessible to protocolize a fluoride vaccine associated with brushing and adequate hygiene in key age groups.

In Manaus, state capital with over 2 million inhabitants, according to IBGE, center of the Amazon rainforest, with acidic water coming from the Rio Negro and its tributaries and without water fluoridation, without basic sanitation and with other problems, with an immense extension, even larger than many European countries, for example, without road access in the state capital, when we go to the interior this multiplies exponentially. Residents of remote areas who only see dentists once every 5 years, where they perform multiple tooth extractions.

I was able to witness the entire catastrophic chain that the lack of water fluoridation in the city of Manaus and the diet based on simple carbohydrates, flour and derivatives cause. Extremely sad, excruciating, painful and that amputates people abruptly and unnecessarily due to the lack of resources, both financial and educational.

When a child does not brush their teeth and starts to develop cavities, this will generate an infection in the mouth, linked to painful symptoms and a decrease in immunity and cognitive capacity. In this way, in the vast majority of cases, the child will be harmed and the possibly infected baby teeth will pass on cavities to the permanent teeth, which appear at 6 years of age on average worldwide, but in hot environments there is scientific evidence that this tooth appears up to 4 years of age.

Parents of all ages and socioeconomic levels do not realize that this tooth is permanent and the child will be crippled for the rest of his or her life if he or she loses it.

Everything could be avoided if there were brushing with fluoride and drinking water with an adequate amount of fluoride.

Thus, water fluoridation at treatment plants has been mandatory in Brazil since 1974, according to Federal Law No. 6,050 /19741, which to this day has not been put into practice and generates billions of reais in financial and psychological losses, as not having teeth changes a person's life forever.

not be able to feed themselves, bite correctly, causing headaches, among other pathologies.

5.7 Protocol for the use of glass ionomer cement in caries

An extremely viable and possible proposal for applying fluoride in a common vaccination method as practiced around the world would be:

Every 6 months, plan visits to the dentist for all children aged 2 and older, with prophylaxis and application of topical fluoride. With delivery of brushing kits with fluoridated toothpaste and dental floss.

And annually apply type R glass ionomer cement, in the plastic phase, obviously performed by a professional dental surgeon on a tooth surface without cavities or with small or inactive cavities, white or darkened, without cavitation.

The advantage of type R (restored) glass ionomer cement is its gradual deposition of fluoride in the area where it is housed, mainly in the occlusal pits and cicatricles of permanent or deciduous molars and in permanent premolars when they erupt.

If we have to renew the flu vaccine every year, why not adopt this method that would bring indelible improvements in the prevalence levels not only of cavities, but also of periodontal disease, would reduce toothaches, work absenteeism, in addition to billions of dollars in dental treatments that could be avoided.

Glass ionomer cement can be replaced by another product with proven efficacy, which is silver diaminefluoride (SDF), a topical application product that combines the remineralization action of fluoride with the bactericidal action of silver, allowing it to act both in the prevention and treatment of caries lesions. Such as Riva Star (SDI Australia), which is a Silver Diamine Fluoride solution system, used to immediately desensitize toothache. Used for over 50 years in Dentistry. This treatment with state-of-the-art SDF enables a minimally invasive technique, whose philosophy is prevention, remineralization and less invasive procedures. Effective biofilm inhibitor.

The silver fluoride and potassium iodide present in Riva Star solution block the microscopic tubules that make up dentin. A low-solubility precipitate is formed, providing instant relief from sensitivity.

Unlike other silver fluoride systems that stain teeth, which does not happen with R-type glass ionomer cements that have other colors, even close to tooth enamel, the two-step Riva Star procedure minimizes the risk of staining. By applying the potassium iodide (KI) solution over the silver diamine fluoride (SDF), a creamy white precipitate of silver iodide is formed and becomes transparent.

Studies confirm that Riva Star (SDI) is an effective biofilm inhibitor. Riva Star has higher zones of inhibition against four bacterial species (E.faecalis, S.gordonni, S.mutans, S.mitis) compared to sodium hypochlorite.

Therefore, we now have the possibility of products with excellent effects: ionomer does not stain and releases fluoride gradually, which is the best in my opinion. However, we also have **silver diaminefluoride** (SDF), which is excellent, but stains the enamel, leaving it grayish. Currently, this solution of potassium iodide (KI) on silver diaminefluoride (SDF), which seems to be excellent, but has not yet reached the global dental market. Therefore, it is cheaper and easier to find glass ionomer cement type R. This is, consequently, the Gold Standard.

Taking into account the total lack of preparation of public policies associated with water fluoridation in adequate proportions and with care in the amount of fluoride applied so as not to cause fluorosis, a pathology that causes stains, generally whitish, that appear on the teeth due to excess fluoride, generally in a symmetrical manner. It generally affects children aged 0 to 12 years in regions where water is fluoridated without control, and has a natural fluoride level greater than 4mg/L (which is very high) in workers in the fluoride industry.

6

VOLUNTEER WORK AND DENTISTRY

Volunteering for healthcare professionals, specifically dentists, has a significant impact on both the community and the professionals themselves. Dentistry, as a health area directly linked to quality of life, finds in volunteering a way to promote oral health, prevent diseases and educate the population about the importance of ongoing care.

6.1 Importance of Volunteering in Dentistry

1. Access to Basic Care: In many underserved communities, access to quality dental care is limited or nonexistent. Volunteer dentists working in social projects provide essential treatments, such as fillings, extractions, and cleanings, that can prevent serious oral health problems. Volunteering, in this sense, acts as a means of social justice, reducing disparities in oral health.

2. Prevention of Oral Diseases: One of the greatest benefits of volunteering in dentistry is the promotion of prevention. Many oral diseases, such as cavities, gingivitis and periodontitis, are preventable with proper hygiene habits and regular visits to the dentist. Volunteer programs often include awareness campaigns, educational lectures and the distribution of oral hygiene kits (toothbrushes, toothpaste, dental floss), empowering people to take care of their own oral health.

3. Oral Health Education: A crucial aspect of prevention is education. Volunteer dentists have the opportunity to teach oral hygiene practices such as proper brushing and flossing, and the importance of a balanced diet to maintain healthy teeth. In many underserved areas, lack of knowledge about these practices contributes to the high incidence of dental problems.

4. Community Strengthening: Volunteer dentists help create a culture of health within the communities they serve. By providing ongoing

care, guidance, and support, professionals help build a network of care, encouraging self-care and mutual support among residents.

5. Benefits for the Professional: In addition to benefiting communities, volunteering offers dentists an opportunity for personal and professional development. By dealing with different contexts and challenges, professionals expand their technical and interpersonal skills. In addition, volunteering provides a deep sense of personal fulfillment by contributing to improving people's lives.

In this way, volunteer work for dentists is a powerful tool for social transformation and public health promotion. By working to promote prevention in dentistry, dentists not only help treat diseases, but also prevent them from occurring, empowering communities to maintain their oral health independently and effectively.

In our experience, we have had moments of great happiness, helping refugees from countries like Haiti and Venezuela, children with limited financial resources, whose parents cannot afford to buy oral hygiene products, children and adults with physical disabilities, such as wheelchair users and paraplegics, patients with Down syndrome, among other conditions, public school students in the state of Amazonas, and people far from large capitals like Manaus. Working with the elderly and indigenous people has been fantastic and has made us more human and more aware of our real role in this world, which we are just passing through, which is to be able to contribute to other people in order to improve their lives in some way. After all, not everything can be bought with money. A smile from a grateful child who knows how to brush their teeth and coincidentally this will change their quality of life and their reality in the world in which they are inserted forever.

In this way, we can see the voluntary activities carried out by us in the following photographs.

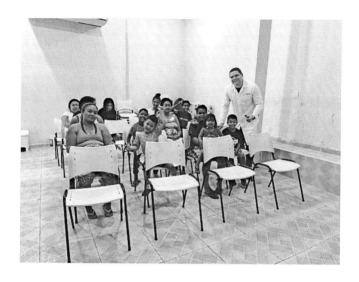

Photo 1. Volunteer work carried out with refugees from Venezuela - Fundação Nascer in Manaus

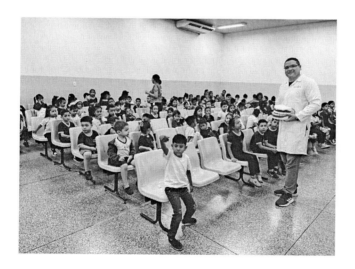

Photo 2. Volunteer work carried out with children aged 4 to 7 at Colégio Odete Barbosa in Manaus

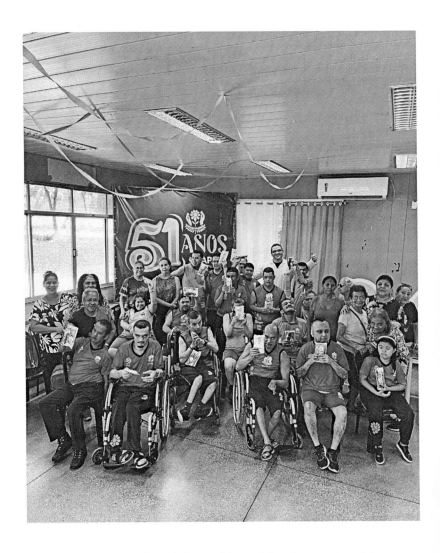

Photo 3. Volunteer work carried out with special patients at Apae Manaus

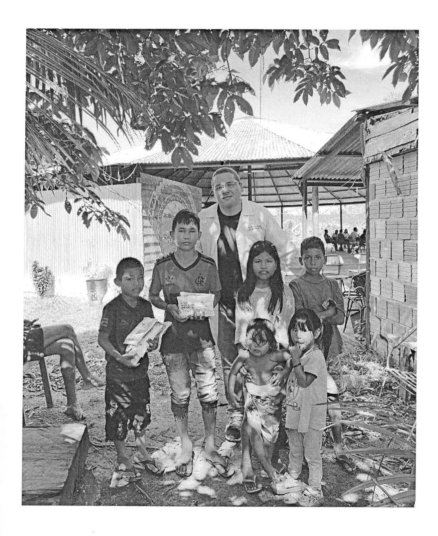

Photo 4. Volunteer work carried out with indigenous children at the Maloca dos Povos Indígenas – Manaus-AM

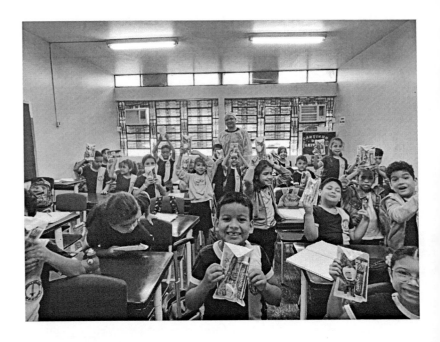

Photo 5. Volunteer work carried out with children aged 6 to 9 at Colegio Major Silva in Manaus

7

CONCLUSION

We conclude that fluoride is indeed an effective and inexpensive measure to prevent tooth decay, changing lives, and can change even more, by drastically reducing tooth decay, the third most prevalent disease in the world. A serious protocol with scientific and clinical basis should be adopted, such as the one we propose, developed with more than 75 years of experience in Dentistry, carried out in an academic manner associated with direct dental practice with patients from all corners of the globe, of all ages and socioeconomic classes, from the poorest refugee from other countries to the richest, all having something in common: the experience of tooth decay that is or has been present in their body at some point in their life, being one of the three most frequent pathologies in the world. Exposing the real need to improve awareness of the disease as a possible cause of worsening of the most diverse diseases, including chronic ones. And with the real creation of a global campaign, Black March, with teaching of oral health techniques and application of prevention techniques, such as restored glass ionomer cement, as an atraumatic sealant, in children under 5, 6 and 7 years old, extending to other ages if necessary, and also topical fluoride and prophylaxis and other dental treatments if necessary. Without bias from financial or sensationalist aspects, which report that fluoride is not necessary, this distorts the scientific truth, to sell more scientific articles or more products that will only generate money for large corporations and harm human beings. Highlighting the absolute need for a responsible and direct public policy. And not the search for an injectable vaccine for cavities, because we have fluoride that when used correctly will prevent in a fantastic way. This work was carried out in order to help and collaborate with the people and for the people of our world. Generating well-being and quality of life, without pain and infection, we therefore affirm that fluoride, when properly applied with a sealant protocol with restorative glass ionomer cement, together with water fluoridation and toothpaste with fluoride, can indeed be the long-awaited vaccine against cavities. It is simple, effective and replicable throughout the world.

REFERENCES

Albuquerque, S. L., Correia Lima, M. G. G., & Sampaio, F. C.. *Evaluation of the use of fluoridated toothpastes in preschool children in the city of João Pessoa - Paraíba - Brazil*. Clinical-Scientific Dentistry. 2003; 2(3): 211-216.

Amarante, L. M. Topical application of fluoride by the mouthwash method. *Rev Bras Odontol*. 1983; 40(4): 23-37.

American Dental Association Council on Scientific Affairs. Professionally applied topical fluoride: Evidence-based clinical recommendations. *J.Am. Dent Assoc*. 2006; 137(8): 1151-9.

Andrade, MF, Moroni, JR, Candido, MSM, & Lofdredo, LCM Effect of fluoride application on surface hardness of glass ionomer cements. *Rev. Assoc. Paul. Cir. Dent*. 1996; 5(2): 193- 96.

Barros, LA, Lopes, FF, Oliveira, AEF, & Ribeiro, CCC Oral fluoride retention after professional topical application in children with caries activity: comparison of fluoride foam and fluoride gel at 1.23%. *RGO*, Porto Alegre. 2008; 56(3): 281-285.

Basting, RT, Pereira, AC, & Meneghim, MC Evaluation of the Prevalence of Dental Caries in Schoolchildren in the Municipality of Piracicaba, SP, Brazil, after 25 years of fluoridation in Brazil. *Journal of Dentistry of the University of São Paulo*. 1997; 11(4): 287-292.

Bijella, MFTB, Brighenti, FL, Bijella, MFB, & Buzalaf, MA R. Fluoride kinetics in saliva after the use of a fluoride-containing chewing gum. *Braz Oral Res*. 2005; 19(4): 256-60.

Bleicher, L., & Frota, F. Water fluoridation: a public policy issue – the case of the State of Ceará. *Science and Public Health*. 2006; 11(1): 71-78.

Brazil, Ministry of Health. *Federal Law No. 6050 of May 24, 1974*. Provides for the fluoridation of water in supply systems when there is a treatment plant, Brasília DF, DO U, 1974.

Brazil, Ministry of Health. *More health in children's smiles*. Health Report, n. 72, Nov. 1998.

Brazil, Ministry of Health. Secretariat of Health Care. Department of Primary Care. National Coordination of Oral Health. *Guidelines for the National Oral Health Policy*. Brasília: Ministry of Health, 2004.

Brazil, Ministry of Health. Secretariat of Health Care. Department of Primary Care. *Guide to recommendations for the use of fluorides in Brazil*. Ministry of Health, Secretariat of Health Care, Department of Primary Care. Brasília: Ministry of Health, 2009.

Brazil, Ministry of Health. *Opinion on Bill No. 510/03*. Provides against the repeal of Law No. 6050/74. Retrieved on December 2, 2015, from http://dtr2001.saude.gov.br/sps/arestecnicas/bucal/home.htm.

Brazil, Ministry of Health. Guidelines for the National Oral Health Policy. Retrieved December 1, 2015, from http://www.saude.gov.br/.

Campos, D. L. *et al.* Prevalence of dental fluorosis in schoolchildren in Brasilia – Federal District. *Dental Journal of the University of São Paulo.* 1998; 12(3): 225-230.

Cangussu, MCT, & Costa, MCN Topical fluoride in the reduction of dental caries in adolescents in Salvador - BA, 1996. *Res. Odontol. Brás.* 2001; 15(4): 348-353.

Cardoso, L. *et al.* Caries polarization in a municipality without fluoridated water. *Cad. Public Health.* 2003; 19(1): 237-243.

Chankanka, O., Levy, SM, Warren, JJ, & Chalmers, JM A literature review of aesthetic perceptions of dental fluorosis and relationships with psychosocial aspects / oral health-related quality of life. *Community Dent Oral Epidemiol.* 2010; 38: 97 - 109.

Chedid, SJ *Evaluation of the amount of fluoridated dentifrice or 0.02% NaF on the development of caries in deciduous teeth:* in vitro study using a pH cycling model [doctoral thesis]. São Paulo: Faculty of Dentistry of the University of São Paulo, 1999.

Choi AL, Sun G, Zhang Y, Grandjean P. Developmental fluoride neurotoxicity: a systematic review and meta-analysis. Environ Health Perspect. doi: 10.1289/

ehp.1104912. Epub 2012 Jul 20. PMID: 22820538; PMCID: PMC3491930. 2012 Oct; 120(10):1362-8.

Cury, J. Use of fluoride. *In* Baratieri, L.N. *Dentistry:* preventive and restorative procedures. 2nd ed. Rio de Janeiro: Quintessence, 1992.

Cury, J. A. *et al.* The importance of fluoride dentifrices to the current dental caries prevalence in Brazil. *Brazilian Dental Journal.* 2004; 15(3): 167-174.

Cury, JA, Narvai, PC, & Castellanos, RA *Recommendations on the use of fluorinated products within the scope of the SUS -SP according to the risk of dental caries.* Dentistry in Public Health: Student Manual. Faculty of Dentistry, University of São Paulo, 2007.

Cypriano, S.S. *et al.* Oral health of schoolchildren living in areas with or without fluoridation in public water supplies in the region of Sorocaba. São Paulo, Brazil. *Public Health Journal.* 2003; 19(4): 1063-1071.

De Almeida, MEC *et al.* Knowledge about fluoride among pediatricians and pediatric dentists in Manaus. Conscientiae Health. 2007; 6(2): 361-369.

Delbem, ACB, Tiano, GC, Alves, KMRP, & Cunha, R. F. Anticariogenic potential of acidulate solutions with low fluoride concentration. *J appl oral sci.* 2006; 14(4): 233-7.

Felix, MCC *et al.* Protective action of fluoride mouthwashes on enamel: in vitro study. *R. Ci. med. biol.* 2004; 3(2): 201-217.

Fjerskov, O., Manji, F., Baelum, V., & Moller, I. J. *Dental Fluorosis:* A Handbook for Health Professionals. São Paulo: Editora Santos, 1994.

Fejerskov, O. Changing paradigms in concepts on dental caries: consequences for oral health care. *Caries Res.* 2004; 38: 182-91.

Frazão, P., Peverari, AC, Forni, & TIB Dental fluorosis: comparison of two prevalence studies. *Cad. Public Health.* 2004; 20(4): 1050-1058.

Garcia, AL Cavities incidence and costs of preventive programs. *J Public Health Dent* 1989; 49: 259-71.

Gomes, P.R. *et al.* Paulínia, São Paulo, Brazil: situation of dental caries in relation to the WHO targets for 2000 and 2010. *Public Health Journal.* 2004; 20(3): 866-870.

Grandjean P. Developmental fluoride neurotoxicity: an updated review. Environ Health. doi: 10.1186/s12940-019-0551-x. PMID: 31856837; PMCID: PMC6923889. 2019 Dec 19;18 (1):110.

Guan, Z. Research into the DNA and RNA content of the cerebellum of chronically fluoride poisoned rats. *J Guizhou Medical College,* 1987; 12(1): 104.

Harari, SG Clinical and pathological features of caries disease. *ABOPREV.* 1996; 7(1): 8-10.

He, H., Cheng, Z., & Liu, W. Effects of fluorine on the human fetus. *Fluoride.* 41(4) 321-326. oct.-dec. 2008.

Hellwig, E., & Lennon, A. M. Systemic versus Topical Fluoride. *Caries Res.* 2004; 38(1): 258-262.

Hoffmann, RHS *et al.* Dental cavities in children at public and private schools from a city with fluoridated water. *Public Health Notebook.* 2004; 20(2): 522-528.

Hortense, P., & Souza, FAEF Comparative scaling of different nociceptive and neuropathic pains through varied psychophysical methods. *Rev Latino-am Enfermagem.* Mar. -Apr. 2009; 17(2). Retrieved June 1, 2023, from www.eerp. usp.br/rlae.

Huo, D. Further observation of radiological changes of endemic food-borne skeletal fluorosis. *Fluoride.* 1984; 17(1): 9-14.

I BGE, Research Directorate, Department of Population and Social Indicators. *National Basic Sanitation Survey* – PNSB, 2000.

Kramer, P. F. *et al. Oral health promotion in pediatric dentistry.* São Paulo: Artes Médicas, 1997.

Kwon, YR., Son KJ., Pandit, S., Kim, JE., Chang, KW., & Jeon, JG. Bioactivity-guided separation of anti-acidogenic substances against Streptococcus mutans UA159 from Polygonum cuspidatum. *Oral Diseases.* 2010; 16: 204-209.

Lacerda, JT, Traebert, J., & Zambenedetti, ML Orofacial pain and absenteeism in workers in the metallurgical and mechanical industries. *Health soc.* 2008; 17(4): 234-238.

Lima, FG *et al.* Twenty-four months of external control of the fluoridation of public water supplies in Pelotas. Rio Grande do Sul, Brazil. *Public Health Journal.* 2004; 20(2): 422-429.

Liporoni, PCS Fluoride & caries. *ABOPREV.* 1995; 6(1): 8-12.

Lodi, CS, Ramires, I., Buzalaf, MAR, & Bastos, JR M. Fluoride concentration in water at the area supplied by the water treatment station of Bauru, SP. *J Appl Oral Sci.* 2006; 14(5): 365-70.

Maia, LC, & Valença, AMG Remineralization of incipient carious lesions in human enamel-case report. *Rev. ABO Nac.* 1995; 2(6): 419-421.

Maia, LC *et al.* Operational control of water fluoridation in Niterói, Rio de Janeiro, Brazil. *Public Health Journal.* 2003; 19(1): 61-67.

Marthaler, TM Successes and drawbacks in the cavities preventive use of fluorides – lessons to be learned from history. *Oral Health Prev Dent.* 2003; 1: 129-40.

Menezes, LM *et al.* Self-perception of fluorosis due to exposure to fluoride through water and toothpaste. *Public Health Journal.* 2002; 36(6): 752-754.

Midorikawa, ET *Dentistry as occupational health as a new professional specialty:* definition of the field of activity and functions of the dentist in the occupational health team. 2000. Dissertation [Master in Dental Sciences] – Faculty of Dentistry, University of São Paulo, São Paulo, 2000.

Ministry of Health. *Survey of Oral Health Conditions of the Brazilian Population –* SB – Brazil 2003. Retrieved on January 5, 2010, from http://portal.saude.gov.br/portal/aplicacoes/busca/busca.cfm.

Modesto, A., & Primo, LG Atraumatic restorative treatment. *ABOPREV.* 1996; 7(1): 12-16.

Mondelli, RF *et al.* Influence of topical fluoride application on the surface of a glazed and polished porcelain. *J Bras Clin Odontol Int.* 2004; 8(44): 148-52.

Murray, J. Basis for the prevention of oral diseases. São Paulo: Editora Santos; 1992.

Noronha, T. P. Influence of fluoride on public health and worker's health – Literature review. Public Policy & Cities Journal, 2024, 13 (2), e1267. https://doi.org/10.23900/2359-1552v13n2-288-2024

Noronha, TP, & Monteiro, JB Morpho-anatomic-chemical study of medicinal plants: Cissus sicyoides and Momordica charantia, Amazon plants with hypoglycemic effect. Journal of Social and Environmental Management, 2024, 18 (11), e09453. https://doi.org/10.24857/rgsa.v18n11-136

Noronha, TP, & Parente, F. Impact of dental health education on quality of life, cost reduction and global economic sustainability. Observatório de la Economía Latinoamericana, 22 (11), 2024.

Novais, R. *et al.* Caries-Sugar Disease Relationship: Prevalence in Children. *Pesq Bras Odontoped Clin Integr.* 2004; 4(3): 199-203.

Nunes, TVFC *et al.* Aspects of water fluoridation and fluorosis – literature review. *Clin.- Cientif. Dentistry.* 2004; 3(2): 97-101.

Oliveira, ER In vivo study of the effect of a pre-brushing mouthwash on the inhibition of neoformation and removal of dental plaque. Master's thesis. São Paulo: School of Dentistry, University of São Paulo, 1996.

Pelletier, AR Maintenance of optimal fluoride levels in public water systems. *J Public Health Dent.* 2004; 64: 237-9.

Ramires, I., Buzalaf, MAR Fluoridation of public water supply and its benefits in controlling dental caries - fifty years in Brazil. *Science and Health.* 2007; 12(4): 1057-1065.

Ripa, LW A half-century of community water fluoridation in the United States: review and commentary. *J Public Health Dent* 1993; 53: 17-44.

Rivka Green, MA, Bruce Lanphear, Richard Hornung *et al.* David Flora, E. Angeles Martinez-Mier, Raichel Neufeld, Pierre Ayotte, Gina Muckle, Christine Till. Association Between Maternal Fluoride Exposure During Pregnancy and IQ Scores in Offspring in Canada. *JAMA Pediatr* 2019.

Rouxel, P., Baglione, M., Loivos, C., & Groisman, S. Topical fluorides: how and when to use them. *PerioNews Journal*. 2008; 2(3): 225-30.

Sales-Peres, SHC *et al.* An epidemiological profile of dental caries in 12 year-old children residing in cities with and without fluoridated water supply in the central western area of the State of Sao Paulo, Brazil. *Public Health Notebook*. 2002; 18(5): 1281-1288.

Santa Catarina. State Law No. 6065/1982. Provides guidelines for fluoridation of public water supply in the state of Santa Catarina. May 24, 1982.

São Paulo. Health Department of the State of São Paulo. Resolution SS-250, dated 08/15/1995. *Official Gazette of the State of São Paulo,* section 1, p. 11, August 1995.

Schuller, AA, & Kalsbeek, H. Effect of the routine professional application of topical fluoride on caries and treatment experience in adolescents of low socio-economic status in the Netherlands. *Res cavities*. 2003; 37(1): 172-177.

Schneider Filho, DA, Prado, IT, Narvai, PC, & Barbosa, SE *Water fluoridation*. How to carry out health surveillance? Rio de Janeiro: Rede Cedros, 1992.

Silva, BB, & Maltz, M. P *revalence of caries, gingivitis and fluorosis in 12-year-old schoolchildren from Porto Alegre – RS, Brazil, 1998/1999*. Brazilian Dental Research. 2001; 15(3): 208-214.

Silva, JS *et al.* Heterocontrol of water fluoridation in three cities in Piauí, Brazil. *Public Health Journal*. 2007; 23(5): 1083-1088.

Silva, MCC *et al.* Effect of fluoridated water on dental caries and fluorosis in schoolchildren who use fluoridated dentifrice. *Braz Dent J.* 2021 may, 32(3): 75-83. Retrieved June 1, 2023, from https://doi.org/10.1590/0103-6440202104167.

Soares, JMP, & Valença, AM G. Clinical Evaluation of the Therapeutic Potential of Fluoride Gel and Veniz. *Pesq Bras Odontoped Clin Integr*. 2003; 3(2): 35-41.

Ten Cate, JM, & van Duinen, RNB Hypermineralization of dentinal lesions adjacent to glass-ionomer cement restorations. *J. Dent. Res.* 1995; 6(74): 1266-71.

Ten Cate, JM Fluorides in Cavities Prevention and Control: Empiricism or Science. *Caries Res.* 2004; 38(1): 254-257.

Tenuta, LMA, Del Bel Cury, AA, Tabchoury, COM, Moi, GP, Silva, WJ, & Cury, J. Á. Kinetics of Monofluorophosphate Hydrolysis in a Bacterial Test Plaque in situ. *Caries Res.* 2010; 44: 55 - 59.

Vilhena, FV *et al.* New protocol for collective oral health actions: standardization in the storage, distribution and use of oral hygiene material. *Ciênc. collective health.* 2008; 13(2): 132-137.

Villena, RS, & Ando, T. Transverse technique for placement of fluoride tooth-paste: an alternative for preschool children. *In Meeting of the Brazilian Society of Dental Research, SBPqO 12.*